Paramedic Care

Principles & Practice

Patient Assessment

Workbook

Third Edition

ROBERT S. PORTER

BRYAN E. BLEDSOE, DO, FACEP, EMT-P

Emergency Physician
Midlothian, Texas
and
Professor, Health Sciences
University of Nevada, Las Vegas
Las Vegas, Nevada

ROBERT S. PORTER, MA, NREMT-P

Senior Advanced Life Support Educator
Madison County Emergency Medical Services
Canastota, New York
and
Flight Paramedic
AirOne, Onondaga County Sheriff's Department
Syracuse, New York

RICHARD A. CHERRY, MS, NREMT-P

Clinical Assistant Professor of Emergency Medicine
Technical Director for Medical Simulation
Upstate Medical University
Syracuse, New York

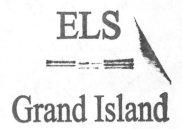

ELS

Grand Island

D1377323

PEARSON
Prentice Hall

Upper Saddle River, New Jersey 07458

Publisher: *Julie Levin Alexander*
Publisher's Assistant: *Regina Bruno*
Executive Editor: *Marlene McHugh Pratt*
Senior Managing Editor for Development: *Lois Berlowitz*
Project Manager: *Triple SSS Press Media Development, Inc.*
Editorial Assistant: *Sean Karpowicz*
Director of Marketing: *Karen Allman*
Executive Marketing Manager: *Katrin Beacom*
Marketing Specialist: *Michael Sirinides*
Managing Editor for Production: *Patrick Walsh*
Production Liaison: *Faye Gemmellaro*
Production Editor: *DeAnn Montoya/S4Carlisle Publishing Services*
Manufacturing Manager: *Ilene Sanford*
Manufacturing Buyer: *Pat Brown*
Senior Design Coordinator: *Christopher Weigand*
Cover Design: *Jill Little*
Cover Image: *Ray Kemp/911 Imaging*
Composition: *S4Carlisle Publishing Services*
Printer/Binder: *Bind-Rite Graphics*
Cover Printer: *Phoenix Color*

NOTICE ON CPR AND ECC

The national standards for Cardiopulmonary Resuscitation (CPR) and Emergency Cardiovascular Care (ECC) are reviewed and revised on a regular basis and may change slightly after this manual is printed. It is important that you know the most current procedures for CPR and ECC, both for the classroom and your patients. The most current information may always be downloaded from www.bradybooks.com or obtained from the appropriate credentialing agency.

NOTICE ON CARE PROCEDURES

It is the intent of the authors and publisher that this Workbook be used as part of a formal EMT-Paramedic program taught by qualified instructors and supervised by a licensed physician. The procedures described in this Workbook are based upon consultation with EMT and medical authorities. The authors and publisher have taken care to make certain that these procedures reflect currently accepted clinical practice; however, they cannot be considered absolute recommendations.

The material in this Workbook contains the most current information available at the time of publication. However, federal, state, and local guidelines concerning clinical practices, including, without limitation, those governing infection control and universal precautions, change rapidly. The reader should note, therefore, that the new regulations may require changes in some procedures.

It is the responsibility of the reader to familiarize himself or herself with the policies and procedures set by federal, state, and local agencies as well as the institution or agency where the reader is employed. The authors and the publisher of this Workbook disclaim any liability, loss, or risk resulting directly or indirectly from the suggested procedures and theory, from any undetected errors, or from the reader's misunderstanding of the text. It is the reader's responsibility to stay informed of any new changes or recommendations made by any federal, state, and local agency as well as by his or her employing institution or agency.

Copyright © 2009 by Pearson Education, Inc., Upper Saddle River, New Jersey 07458. Pearson Prentice Hall. All rights reserved. Printed in the United States of America. This publication is protected by Copyright and permission should be obtained from the publisher prior to any prohibited reproduction, storage in a retrieval system, or transmission in any form or by any means, electronic, mechanical, photocopying, recording, or likewise. For information regarding permission(s), write to: Rights and Permissions Department.

Pearson Prentice Hall™ is a trademark of Pearson Education, Inc.
Pearson® is a registered trademark of Pearson plc.
Prentice Hall® is a registered trademark of Pearson Education, Inc.

Pearson Education Ltd., London
Pearson Education Singapore, Pte. Ltd.
Pearson Education Canada, Inc.
Pearson Education—Japan
Pearson Education Australia Pty. Limited
Pearson Education North Asia, Ltd., Hong Kong
Pearson Educación de Mexico, S.A. de C.V.
Pearson Education Malaysia, Pte. Ltd.
Pearson Education, Upper Saddle River, New Jersey

10 9 8 7 6 5 4 3 2
ISBN: 0-13-515071-X
ISBN: 978-0-13-515071-9

Dedication

To Kris and sailing: pleasant distractions from teaching, writing about, and practicing prehospital emergency medicine.

CONTENTS

INTRODUCTION

Welcome to the self-instructional Workbook for *Paramedic Care: Principles & Practice*, Third Edition. This Workbook is designed to help guide you through an educational program for initial or refresher training that follows the guidelines of the 1998 U.S. Department of Transportation EMT-Paramedic National Standard Curriculum. The Workbook is designed to be used either in conjunction with your instructor or as a self-study guide you use on your own.

This Workbook features many different ways to help you learn the material necessary to become a paramedic.

Features

Review of Chapter Objectives

Each chapter of *Paramedic Care: Principles & Practice* begins with objectives that identify the important information and principles addressed in the chapter reading. To help you identify and learn this material, each Workbook chapter reviews the important content elements addressed by these objectives as presented in the text.

Case Study Review

Each chapter of *Paramedic Care: Principles & Practice* includes a case study, introducing and highlighting important principles presented in the chapter. The Workbook reviews these case studies and points out much of the essential information and many of the applied principles they describe.

Content Self-Evaluation

Each chapter of *Paramedic Care: Principles & Practice* presents an extensive narrative explanation of the principles of paramedic practice. The Workbook chapter (or chapter section) contains between 10 and 50 multiple-choice questions to test your reading comprehension of the textbook material and to give you experience taking typical emergency medical service examinations.

Special Projects

The Workbook contains several projects that are special learning experiences designed to help you remember the information and principles necessary to perform as a paramedic. Special projects include crossword puzzles, fill in the blank, and a variety of other exercises.

Prehospital Care Reports

The Workbook provides you with narrative information regarding simulated calls and then asks you to record that information on prehospital care report forms. These exercises help you refine your abilities to identify important medical information and record it on the prehospital care reports as you would in real life.

Personal Benchmarking

The Workbook provides several exercises that direct you to evaluate elements of the patient assessment process on yourself. These exercises help you develop your assessment skills and use normal findings as benchmarks for reference when you begin your career as a paramedic.

Chapter Sections

Several chapters in *Paramedic Care: Principles & Practice* are extensive and contain a great deal of subject matter. To help you grasp this material more efficiently, the Workbook breaks these chapters into sections with their own objectives, content review, and special projects.

Content Review

The Workbook provides a comprehensive review of the material presented in this volume of *Paramedic Care: Principles & Practice*. After the last text chapter has been covered, the Workbook presents an extensive content self-evaluation component that helps you recall and build upon the knowledge you have gained by reading the text, attending class, and completing the earlier Workbook chapters.

Patient Scenario Flash Cards

At the end of this Workbook are scenario flash cards, which are designed to help you practice the processes of investigating both the chief complaint and the past medical history. Each card contains the dispatch information and results of the scene size-up and then prompts you to inquire into either the patient's major symptoms or past medical history.

©2009 Pearson Education, Inc.
Paramedic Care: Principles & Practice, Vol. 2, 3rd. Ed.

HOW TO USE THIS SELF-INSTRUCTIONAL WORKBOOK

The self-instructional Workbook accompanying *Paramedic Care: Principles & Practice* may be used as directed by your instructor or independently by you during your course of instruction. The following recommendations are intended to guide you in using the Workbook independently.

- Examine your course schedule and identify the appropriate text chapter or other assigned reading.

- Read the assigned chapter in *Paramedic Care: Principles & Practice* carefully. Do this in a relaxed environment, free of distractions, and give yourself adequate time to read and digest the material. The information presented in *Paramedic Care: Principles & Practice* is often technically complex and demanding, but it is very important that you comprehend it. Be sure that you read the chapter carefully enough to understand and remember what you have read.

- Carefully read the Review of Chapter Objectives at the beginning of each Workbook chapter (or section). This material includes both the objectives listed in *Paramedic Care: Principles & Practice* and narrative descriptions of their content. If you do not understand or remember what is discussed from your reading, refer to the referenced pages and reread them carefully. If you still do not feel comfortable with your understanding of any objective, consider asking your instructor about it.

- Reread the case study in *Paramedic Care: Principles & Practice*, and then read the Case Study Review in the Workbook. Note the important points regarding assessment and care that the Case Study Review highlights and be sure that you understand and agree with the analysis of the call. If you have any questions or concerns, ask your instructor to clarify the information.

- Take the Content Self-Evaluation at the end of each Workbook chapter (or section), answering each question carefully. Do this in a quiet environment, free from distractions, and allow yourself adequate time to complete the exercise. Correct your self-evaluation by consulting the answers at the back of the Workbook, and determine the percentage you have answered correctly (the number you got right divided by the total number of questions). If you have answered most of the questions correctly (85 to 90 percent), review those that you missed by rereading the material on the pages listed in the Answer Key and be sure you understand which answer is correct and why. If you have more than a few questions wrong (less than 85 percent correct), look for incorrect answers that are grouped together. This suggests that you did not understand a particular topic in the reading. Reread the text dealing with that topic carefully, and then retest yourself on the questions you got wrong. If incorrect answers are spread throughout the chapter content, reread the chapter and retake the Content Self-Evaluation to ensure that you understand the material. If you don't understand why your answer to a question is incorrect after reviewing the text, consult with your instructor.

- In a similar fashion, complete the exercises in the Special Projects section of the Workbook chapters (or sections). These exercises are specifically designed to help you learn and remember the essential principles and information presented in *Paramedic Care: Principles & Practice*.

- When you have completed this volume of *Paramedic Care: Principles & Practice* and its accompanying Workbook, prepare for a course test by reviewing both the text in its entirety and your class notes. Then take the Content Review examination in the Workbook. Again, review your score and any questions you have answered incorrectly by referring to the text and rereading the page or pages where the material is presented. If you note groupings of wrong answers, review the entire range of pages or the full chapter they represent.

If, during your completion of the Workbook exercises, you have any questions that either the textbook or the Workbook doesn't answer, write them down and ask your instructor about them. Prehospital emergency medicine is a complex and complicated subject, and answers are not always black-and-white. It is also common for different EMS systems to use differing methods of care. The questions you bring up in class, and your instructor's answers to them, will help you expand and complete your knowledge of prehospital emergency medical care.

The authors and Brady Publishing continuously seek to ensure the creation of the best materials to support your educational experience. We are interested in your comments. If, during your reading and study of material in *Paramedic Care: Principles & Practice,* you notice any error or have any suggestions to improve either the textbook or the Workbook, please direct your comments via the Internet to the following address:

hiawatha@localnet.com

You can also visit the Brady website at:
www.bradybooks.com/paramedic

©2009 Pearson Education, Inc.
Paramedic Care: Principles & Practice, Vol. 2, 3rd. Ed.

GUIDELINES TO BETTER TEST-TAKING

The knowledge you will gain from reading the textbook, completing the exercises in the Workbook, listening in your paramedic class, and participating in your clinical and field experience will prepare you to care for patients who are seriously ill or injured. However, before you can practice these skills, you will have to pass several classroom written exams and your state's certification exam. Your performance on these exams will depend not only on your knowledge but also on your ability to answer test questions correctly. The following guidelines are designed to help your performance on tests and to better demonstrate your knowledge of prehospital emergency care.

1. Relax and be calm during the test.

A test is designed to measure what you have learned and to tell you and your instructor how well you are doing. An exam is not designed to intimidate or punish you. Consider it a challenge, and just try to do your best. Get plenty of sleep before the examination. Avoid coffee or other stimulants for a few hours before the exam, and be prepared.

Reread the text chapters, review the objectives in the Workbook, and review your class notes. It might be helpful to work with one or two other students and ask each other questions. This type of practice helps everyone better understand the knowledge presented in your course of study.

2. Read the questions carefully.

Read each word of the question and all the answers slowly. Words such as "except" and "not" change the entire meaning of the question. If you miss such words, you may answer the question incorrectly, even though you know the right answer.

EXAMPLE:
The art and science of emergency medical services involves all of the following EXCEPT:

> A. sincerity and compassion.
> B. respect for human dignity.
> C. placing patient care before personal safety.
> D. delivery of sophisticated emergency medical care.
> E. none of the above.

The correct answer is C, unless you miss the "EXCEPT."

3. Read each answer carefully.

Read every answer carefully. While the first answer may be absolutely correct, so may the rest, and thus the best answer might be "all of the above."

EXAMPLE:
Indirect medical direction is considered to be:

> A. treatment protocols.
> B. training and education.
> C. quality assurance.
> D. chart review.
> E. all of the above.

While answers A, B, C, and D are correct, the best and only acceptable answer is "all of the above," E.

4. Delay answering questions you don't understand and look for clues.

When a question seems confusing or you don't know the answer, note it on your answer sheet and go back to it later. This will ensure that you have time to complete the test. You will also find that other questions in the test may give you hints to answer the one you've skipped over. It will also prevent you from being frustrated with an early question and letting it affect your performance.

EXAMPLE:
Upon successful completion of a course of training as an EMT-P, most states will:

    A. certify you (correct).
    B. license you.
    C. register you.
    D. recognize you as a paramedic.
    E. issue you a permit.

Another question, later in the exam, may suggest the right answer:

The action of one state in recognizing the certification of another called:

    A. reciprocity. (correct)
    B. national registration.
    C. licensure.
    D. registration.
    E. extended practice.

5. Answer all questions.

Even if you do not know the right answer, do not leave a question blank. A blank question is always wrong, while a guess might be correct. If you can eliminate some of the answers as wrong, do so. It will increase the chances of a correct guess.

A multiple-choice question with five answers gives a 20 percent chance of a correct guess. If you can eliminate one or more incorrect answers, you increase your odds of a correct guess to 25 percent, 33 percent, and so on. An unanswered question has a 0 percent chance of being correct.

Just before turning in your answer sheet, check to be sure that you have not left any items blank.

EXAMPLE:
When a paramedic is called by the patient (through the dispatcher) to the scene of a medical emergency, the medical direction physician has established a physician/patient relationship.

    A. True
    B. False

A true/false question gives you a 50 percent chance of a correct guess.

The hospital health professional responsible for sorting patients as they arrive at the emergency department is usually the:

    A. emergency physician.
    B. ward clerk.
    C. emergency nurse.
    D. trauma surgeon.
    E. both A and C. (correct)

©2009 Pearson Education, Inc.
Paramedic Care: Principles & Practice, Vol. 2, 3rd. Ed.

1

The History

Review of Chapter Objectives

With each chapter of the Workbook, we identify the objectives and the important elements of the text content. You should review these items and refer to the pages listed if any points are not clear.

After reading this chapter, you should be able to:

1. Describe the techniques of history taking. **pp. 9–10**

For successful history taking, establish a rapport with the patient to gain his confidence and to set the stage for investigation of the chief complaint and medical history. Factors that will help in establishing rapport include

- Well-groomed initial appearance
- Positive body language
- Good eye contact with the patient
- Professional demeanor
- Demonstration of interest in the patient

Your introduction should demonstrate your interest in helping the patient, begin establishing a rapport, and include obtaining consent to treat. It should convey your care and compassion for the patient and build his trust in you.

Once you have introduced yourself and established your intent to help the patient, begin your questioning. Determine the formal chief complaint and investigate the current and past medical history. Pose questions in a way the patient understands, using terminology and the English language at the patient's level of comprehension.

Questioning frequently involves asking the patient personal, and possibly embarrassing, questions. At such times, ask these questions in a sensitive, nonthreatening way. "Ease into" the discussion of sensitive topics and use questions that are nonjudgmental. You may suggest to the patient that the issue of concern to him is common to many people in our society. Practice in questioning will help you develop the most effective approach. Be prepared to explain that the answers to questions are used for the patient's care and are not communicated beyond the necessary care providers.

2. Discuss the importance of using open- and closed-ended questions. **pp. 6–7**

Open-ended questions allow the patient to explain or describe his symptoms or history in detail. This permits more complete and accurate patient answers and limits possible leading of patient responses.

Closed-ended questions limit patient responses to short answers—"yes" or "no," for example. Their use speeds information taking, but the answers provide only limited information and may lead the patient toward answers.

During a complete patient history, use both types of questions to determine rapidly the nature and severity of the patient's problem and his medical history. Let what the patient tells you guide your questioning process. Focus on the possible medical problem, eliminating the least likely and identifying the most probable pathological condition.

3. **Describe the use of, and differentiate between, facilitation, reflection, clarification, empathetic responses, confrontation, and interpretation.** pp. 8–9

Facilitation is the support and encouragement of the patient as he explains his problem and answers your questions—for example, good eye contact, concerned facial expressions, and leaning forward while listening.

Reflection is condensing and repeating what the patient says, to guide patient response and encourage more focused answers.

Clarification is investigating a patient's response by asking questions about it to garner further, more specific information.

Empathetic responses are facial expressions or statements such as "I see" or "That must have been difficult" that display an understanding of, and a supportive feeling for, the patient's situation.

Confrontation is the questioning of a patient's responses when he appears to be lying about or denying the truth.

Interpretation takes confrontation a step further. You interpret your observations and question your patient about what you believe may be the problem.

4. **Describe the structure, purpose, and how to obtain a comprehensive patient history.** pp. 4–23

The comprehensive health history establishes a relationship between you and the patient and draws out pertinent information about the patient's medical history. This information may explain the current problem or guide further care in either the prehospital or the in-hospital setting. The comprehensive patient history is gained by investigative questioning of the patient about past and current medical problems, including the chief complaint, present illness (onset, provocation/palliation, quality, region/radiation, severity, time, associated symptoms, pertinent negatives [OPQRST-ASPN]), past medical history, and current health status, as well as a review of systems.

5. **List the components of a comprehensive history of an adult patient.** pp. 10–19

The comprehensive patient history includes

- Preliminary data (age, race, sex, and so on)
- Chief complaint
- Present illness or problem (including OPQRST-ASPN)
- Past medical history (including patient's general health, childhood and adult illnesses, psychiatric illnesses, serious accidents or injuries, and surgeries and hospitalizations)
- Current health status (including patient medications; allergies; use of tobacco, drugs, or alcohol; diet; recent screening tests and immunizations; exercise; leisure and sleep patterns; environmental hazard/safety measures; family history; and psychosocial history)
- Review of systems (including, as appropriate, general physical information; skin; head, eyes, ears, nose, and throat (HEENT); respiratory; cardiac; gastrointestinal; urinary; reproductive; peripheral vascular; musculoskeletal; neurologic; hematologic; endocrine; and psychiatric)

The following objectives, while not listed in the chapter, will help in your understanding of the chapter contents.

*Describe the review of systems and explain how it assists in identifying the patient's primary medical problem. pp. 17–19

The review of systems is an examination of each body system during the patient history. It is performed to rule out or further investigate medical problems and to ensure that pertinent information is not overlooked during the assessment. Systems examined include

- Skin
- Head, eyes, ears, nose, throat (HEENT)
- Respiratory
- Cardiac

©2009 Pearson Education, Inc.
Paramedic Care: Principles & Practice, Vol. 2, 3rd. Ed.

- Gastrointestinal
- Urinary
- Reproductive
- Peripheral vascular
- Musculoskeletal
- Neurologic
- Hematologic
- Endocrine
- Psychiatric

*Identify techniques for working with patients with special challenges.   pp. 19–23

Silent patient. Be patient. Speak reassuringly. Gently shake the patient. Consider a neurologic problem.

Overly talkative patient. Focus the patient on important areas. Summarize what he says. Be patient.

Numerous symptoms. Be more clear while questioning; suspect an emotional problem.

Anxious patient. Encourage free conversation and reassure the patient.

Patient needing reassurance. Ask about his anxieties. Offer emotional support.

Angry and hostile patient. Accept the patient's responses without becoming defensive or angry.

Intoxicated patient. Be friendly and nonjudgmental. Listen to what the patient says, not how he says it. Make safety a priority.

Crying patient. Be patient and supportive. Accept the crying as a natural venting of emotions.

Depressed patient. Recognize the condition as a serious medical problem. Ask the patient whether he has had suicidal thoughts.

Sexually attractive or seductive patient. Maintain a professional relationship. Try to have a partner present.

Patient with confusing behaviors or histories. Suspect mental illness, dementia, or delirium. Pay careful attention to the patient's mental status. Be reassuring.

Patient of limited intelligence. Try to evaluate the patient's mental abilities. Show genuine interest and establish a positive relationship. Elicit what information you can.

Language barriers. Seek out an interpreter. Be aware that important information is likely to be lost in translation.

Patient with hearing problems. Speak to the patient's best ear. If he reads lips, position yourself directly in front of him in good lighting, and speak slowly in a low-pitched voice. Consider providing paper for your questions and patient responses.

Patient who is blind or has limited vision. Identify yourself immediately and explain why you are there. Explain what you are going to do before you do it.

Family and friends. If gaining pertinent information directly from the patient is difficult, talk to family members or friends on the scene.

Case Study Review

It is important to review each emergency response you participate in as a paramedic. Similarly, we will review the case study that precedes each chapter. We will address the important points of the response as addressed by the chapter. Often, this will include scene size-up, patient assessment, patient management, patient packaging, and transport.

Reread the case study on pages 2 and 3 in Paramedic Care: Patient Assessment *and then read the discussion following.*

This case study draws attention to the value of the information gathered during the patient history and the process by which it is obtained.

The investigation of the chief complaint, associated symptoms, and past medical history is extremely important both in determining what is wrong with your patient and in guiding your provision of care. The circumstances of the emergency and the patient's presentation may confound you unless you employ a relatively standard, systematic approach to patient questioning. Questioning must remain flexible enough to adapt to different circumstances. In a trauma emergency, you examine the mechanism of injury to determine what happened, whereas with a medical patient you must investigate the current and past medical history in depth.

Paramedic supervisor John Bigelow is presented with an "elderly man with abdominal pain." He begins his investigation of the history by introducing himself, identifying his role at the scene, and expressing his desire to help Mr. O'Donnell. He also asks for and uses Mr. O'Donnell's name to place the conversation on a more comfortable and personal level.

John first determines the patient's chief complaint, the problem that led him to call for the ambulance. (This may differ from the primary problem in some cases.) In this case, the chief complaint is "My stomach hurts." John then quickly investigates the complaint by asking questions. The questions he asks are extensive and systematically examine the patient's symptoms. Note that these questions follow the acronym OPQRST-ASPN. John questions about onset (*What were you doing when it started? Did it come on suddenly?*), provocation/palliation (*Does anything make it better or worse?*), quality (*Can you describe how it feels?*), radiation (*Can you point to the area that hurts? Does the pain travel anywhere else?*), severity (*How bad is it? On a scale of one to ten, with ten being the worst pain you have ever felt, how would you rate this pain?*), time (*When did it start? Is it constant or does it come and go?*), and associated symptoms and pertinent negatives (*Are you nauseous and have you vomited? Have you experienced a change in your bowel habits? Do you have any difficulty breathing?*). As John asks these questions, he leans forward and repeats parts of the patient's answers to show his interest and involvement.

The approach that John uses ensures an ordered and in-depth investigation of all elements of the patient's history. At the emergency scene, there is much going on and often a sense of urgency. However, taking the few moments to inquire systematically about the patient's presentation ensures that you have the essential information to begin forming a differential field diagnosis.

Based on what he has discovered, John begins to form his differential field diagnosis. Although the history of pain immediately after eating suggests gallbladder problems (cholecystitis), John suspects a broader list of potential problems. This keeps him from forming tunnel vision. As he investigates the past medical history, he asks questions to support or rule out these other problems.

John questions Mr. O'Donnell about his past medical history and gains further information about pain after eating fatty foods, indigestion, and alcohol consumption. The patient's denials of bloody emesis and stools are pertinent negatives that help John rule out other possible diagnoses. This information also helps him confirm a final field diagnosis of gallbladder problems. With the facts that support his evaluation, John conveys the results of his patient questioning to Dr. Zehner at the emergency department. The laboratory findings support the field diagnosis, and Mr. O'Donnell is quickly moved to surgery.

Content Self-Evaluation

Each chapter in this Workbook includes a short content review. The questions are designed to test your ability to remember what you have read. At the end of this Workbook, you can find the answers to the questions, as well as the pages where the topic of each question was discussed in the text. If you answer the question incorrectly or are unsure of the answer, review the pages listed.

MULTIPLE CHOICE

_____ 1. In the majority of medical cases, the basis of the paramedic's field diagnosis is the:
   A. chief complaint.
   B. index of suspicion.
   C. mechanism of injury.
   D. patient history.
   E. vital signs.

_____ 2. Always accept information from previous caregivers gratefully, but briefly reconfirm it with the patient.
   A. True
   B. False

©2009 Pearson Education, Inc.
Paramedic Care: Principles & Practice, Vol. 2, 3rd. Ed.

_____ 3. Elements of your patient questioning that will help you establish a trusting and professional relationship with the patient include all of the following EXCEPT:
   A. using medical terminology extensively.
   B. making eye contact.
   C. positioning yourself at the patient's eye level.
   D. presenting a neat and clean appearance.
   E. focusing your attention on the patient.

_____ 4. The list of possible causes for a patient's symptoms is the:
   A. index of suspicion.
   B. mechanism of injury.
   C. differential field diagnosis.
   D. CAGE questionnaire.
   E. nature of illness.

_____ 5. It is appropriate, if not necessary, to take notes while interviewing the patient because it is nearly impossible to remember everything important the patient tells you.
   A. True
   B. False

_____ 6. Which of the following is an example of an open-ended question?
   A. Does your chest pain increase with breathing?
   B. Do you take diuretics?
   C. What does your pain feel like?
   D. Does the pain radiate to your shoulder?
   E. Have you had pain like this before?

_____ 7. Which of the following questions is an example of a closed-ended question?
   A. What does your pain feel like?
   B. What were you doing when the pain started?
   C. Is your pain stabbing in nature?
   D. Why did you call us today?
   E. Where do you hurt?

_____ 8. Always use a patient's first name during the interview to establish a closer, more trusting relationship.
   A. True
   B. False

_____ 9. It is best to form a prearranged list of specific questions to ensure you cover all bases while interviewing your patient.
   A. True
   B. False

_____ 10. The process of presenting the patient with an observation that he is hiding or masking the truth is called:
   A. empathy.
   B. confrontation.
   C. reflection.
   D. clarification.
   E. facilitation.

_____ 11. The reason (pain, discomfort, or dysfunction) that the patient or another person summons emergency medical services is termed the:
   A. primary problem.
   B. chief complaint.
   C. nature of the illness.
   D. mechanism of injury.
   E. none of the above.

_____ 12. The underlying cause of the patient's pain, discomfort, or dysfunction is called the:
   A. primary problem.
   B. chief complaint.
   C. nature of the illness.
   D. mechanism of injury.
   E. none of the above.

_____ 13. Any activity that alleviates a patient's symptoms would fit under which element of the OPQRST-ASPN mnemonic for the history of the current illness?
A. O
B. P
C. Q
D. R
E. S

_____ 14. Which of the following is an important part of the past medical history?
A. radiation of the pain
B. last oral intake
C. surgeries or hospitalizations
D. quality of the pain
E. all of the above

_____ 15. A recently prescribed medication may account for medical problems because of which of the following?
A. overmedication
B. undermedication
C. allergic reaction
D. untoward reaction
E. all of the above

_____ 16. Allergies should be expected for all of the following EXCEPT:
A. the "caine" family.
B. tetanus toxoid.
C. glucose.
D. narcotics.
E. both A and B.

_____ 17. A patient who has smoked 21 packs of cigarettes a week for 10 years has a pack history of:
A. 21 pack/years.
B. 70 pack/years.
C. 7 pack/years.
D. 30 pack/years.
E. 10 pack/years.

_____ 18. Which of the following is NOT a system examined during the review of systems?
A. skin
B. lymphatic system
C. musculoskeletal system
D. hematologic system
E. endocrine system

_____ 19. Which of the following would you attempt with a patient who suddenly goes silent?
A. Stay calm and observe for nonverbal clues.
B. Arrange for air medical transport.
C. Terminate the interview immediately.
D. Attempt to walk the patient back and forth a few times.
E. Rapidly provide oral glucose.

_____ 20. Crying is a form of venting emotional stress; be patient and provide a patient who is crying with supportive remarks.
A. True
B. False

MATCHING

Write the letter of the interview technique in the space provided next to the appropriate description.

_____ 21. Repeating the patient's words

_____ 22. Using "go on" or "I'm listening"

_____ 23. Asking questions about the patient's statements

_____ 24. Showing you understand or feel for the patient

_____ 25. Challenging a patient's statement

A. empathy

B. confrontation

C. reflection

D. facilitation

E. clarification

©2009 Pearson Education, Inc.
Paramedic Care: Principles & Practice, Vol. 2, 3rd. Ed.

Classify each question or statement under the OPQRST category that best applies by writing the letter of the category in the space provided.

O. onset

P. provocation/palliation

Q. quality

R. region/radiation

S. severity

T. time

_____ 26. How does this compare to the worst pain you have ever felt?

_____ 27. Does rest lessen your pain?

_____ 28. Point to where you feel pain.

_____ 29. Does this pain feel crushing in nature?

_____ 30. Does deep breathing increase the pain?

_____ 31. Did this pain begin suddenly or gradually?

_____ 32. Where does this pain travel to?

_____ 33. When did the first symptoms begin?

_____ 34. Describe how the pain feels.

_____ 35. Were you walking or running when this pain first began?

SHORT ANSWER

36. Compare and contrast the differential field diagnosis and the final field diagnosis.

_____

_____

_____

_____

Special Project

History of the Present Illness

Read the following narrative description of a patient history, and then organize the information into the OPQRST-ASPN format.

At just about noon, your unit, Rescue 31, responds to a "man down" call at a local park. You arrive to find an approximately 20-year-old male on the ground surrounded by onlookers. The man is sitting up and talking with a police officer. You introduce yourself and begin to form a general impression of the patient. He is articulate and appears to be conscious, alert, and fully oriented. The patient states that he was jogging when he suddenly had a sharp chest pain, became dizzy, and collapsed. He now complains of mild difficulty breathing and increased pain with deep breathing.

The patient states that the pain is very severe and ranks about 8 on a 1-to-10 scale, with 10 being the worst pain he has ever experienced. He describes the pain as stabbing and indicates its location, which is just to the left of the sternum at about the 3rd intercostal space.

He denies pain anywhere else. The pain began suddenly, without warning, and he has never experienced anything like it. He denies taking a deep breath or coughing before the pain began. He says he has not had previous breathing or chest problems and says he does not have any history of COPD, asthma, or heart problems. He is not currently taking any medications, nor is he being treated for any medical problem.

O. _____

_____

P. _____

_____

Q. _____

_____

R. _____

_____

S. _____

_____

T. _____

_____

AS. _____

_____

PN. _____

_____

©2009 Pearson Education, Inc.
Paramedic Care: Principles & Practice, Vol. 2, 3rd. Ed.

Physical Exam Techniques

Becauase Chapter 2 is lengthy, it has been divided into sections to aid your study. Read the assigned text pages; then progress through the objectives and self-evaluation materials as you would with other chapters. When you feel confident of your grasp of the content, proceed to the next section.

Section I, pp. 27–84

Review of Chapter Objectives

After reading this chapter, you should be able to:

1. Define and describe the techniques of inspection, palpation, percussion, and auscultation. pp. 31–35

Inspection is the process of informed observation, viewing the patient for anatomical shape, coloration, and movement. It is the least invasive examination tool yet may provide the most patient information.

Palpation is the use of touch to gather information regarding size, shape, position, temperature, moisture, texture, movement, and response to pressure. The fingertips are most sensitive, the palm best evaluates vibration, and the back of the hand is most sensitive to temperature.

Percussion is the production of a vibration in tissue to elicit sounds. These sounds—dull, resonant, hyperresonant, tympanic, and flat—identify the nature of the tissue underneath. The vibration is generated by striking the first knuckle of a finger placed against the area to be percussed with the fingertip of the other hand.

Auscultation is listening for sounds within the body, most frequently with a stethoscope. The intensity, pitch, duration, quality, and timing of sounds in the patient's lungs, heart, blood vessels, and intestines are compared against normal sounds.

3. Evaluate the importance of a general survey. pp. 35–51

The general survey is the first part of the comprehensive exam. It is made up of your evaluation of the patient's appearance—including level of consciousness, expression, state of health, general characteristics (for example, weight, height), posturing, dress, grooming, and so on—the vital signs, and additional assessments, such as pulse oximetry, cardiac monitoring, and blood glucose determination. The survey helps you form a general impression of your patient's health.

4. **Describe the examination of the following body regions, differentiate between normal and abnormal findings, and define the significance of abnormal findings.**

Skin, hair, and nails   pp. 60–62

Observe the skin carefully for color, especially in the nail beds, lips, conjunctiva, and mucous membranes of the mouth. Pink skin reflects good oxygenation, whereas pale skin reflects poor blood flow from hypovolemia, hypothermia, compensatory shock, or anemia. A bluish skin, referred to as cyanosis, suggests the blood is low in oxygen. A yellow sclera or general discoloration, termed jaundice, is due to liver failure. Other skin observations may include petechiae, which are small, round, flat, purplish spots caused by capillary bleeding from a variety of etiologies, and ecchymosis, a larger, black-and-blue discoloration that is often the result of trauma or bleeding disorders. Moisture, temperature, texture, mobility, and turgor are also evaluated. Skin lesions are disruptions in normal tissue that may take on almost any shape, color, or arrangement.

Inspect and palpate the hair to determine color, quality, distribution, quantity, and texture and inspect and palpate the scalp for scaling, lesions, redness, lumps, or tenderness. Generalized hair loss may reflect chemotherapy; failure to develop normal hair patterns may be caused by a pituitary or hormonal problem; and unusual facial hair in women suggests a hormonal imbalance. Mild scalp flaking suggests dandruff; heavy scaling, psoriasis; and greasy scaling, seborrheic dermatitis. Lice eggs (nits) may be found firmly attached to the hair shafts. Normal hair texture is smooth and soft in Caucasians; in people of African descent, the texture is coarser. Dry, brittle, or fragile hair is abnormal.

Inspect the fingernails and toenails for color. Note any discolorations, lesions, ridging, grooves, depressions, or pitting. Depressions suggest systemic disease. Compress the nail and bed to determine its adherence and look for nail hygiene. Any boggyness suggests cardiorespiratory disease.

Head, scalp, and skull   pp. 60–62

Observe and palpate the skull and facial region for symmetry, smoothness, wounds, bleeding, size, and general contour. Examine the hair and scalp as described previously. Check the eyes for bilateral periorbital and mastoid ecchymosis, "raccoon eyes" and "Battle's sign," respectively. They suggest basilar skull fracture and occur an hour or so after injury. Palpate the facial region for crepitation, false motion, or instability suggesting fracture. Evaluate the temporomandibular joint for pain, tenderness, swelling, and range of motion. Have the patient open and close his mouth and jut and retract his jaw. Any loss of normal function suggests injury.

Eyes, ears, nose, mouth, and pharynx   pp. 62–82

Examine for visual acuity as described in objective 5; then evaluate for peripheral vision. While the patient faces you, have him look at your nose while you extend your arms, bend your elbows, and wiggle your fingers. If he notices the fingers moving in all four directions (up, down, left, and right) for each eye, his peripheral vision is grossly normal. Inspect the eyes for symmetry, shape, inflammation, swelling, misalignment (disconjugate gaze), lesions, and contour. Examine the eyelids, open and closed, for swelling, discoloration, droop (ptosis), styes, and lash positioning. Observe the tearing or dryness of the eyes. Gently retract the lower eyelid while asking the patient to look through a range of motion. Examine the sclera for signs of irritation, cloudiness, yellow discoloration (jaundice), any nodules, swelling, discharge, or hemorrhage into the scleral tissue. With an oblique light source, inspect the cornea for opacities. Inspect the size, shape, symmetry, and reactivity of the pupils. Note the pupils' direct and consensual response to increased light intensity. A sluggish pupil suggests pressure on CN-III; bilateral sluggishness suggests global hypoxia or depressant drug action. Constricted pupils suggest opiate overdose; dilated and fixed pupils reflect brain anoxia. Ask the patient to focus on your finger close at hand; then move the hand to his nose, then away. The eyes should converge, and the pupils should constrict slightly. Then have him follow your finger as you move it through an "H" pattern. The eyes should move smoothly together. Nystagmus is a jerky movement at the distal extremes of ocular movement. Gently touch the cornea with a strand of cotton. The patient should respond with a blink. Using an ophthalmoscope, look into the eye's anterior chamber for signs of blood (hyphema), cells, or pus (hypopyon) and check the cornea for lacerations, abrasions, cataracts, papilledema (from increased intracranial pressure), vascular occlusions, and retinal hemorrhage.

©2009 Pearson Education, Inc.
Paramedic Care: Principles & Practice, Vol. 2, 3rd. Ed.

Examine the ears by looking for symmetry from in front of the patient; then examine each ear separately. Examine the external portion (auricle) for shape, size, landmarks, and position on the head. Examine the surrounding area for deformities, lesions, tenderness, and erythema. Pull the helix upward and outward, press on the tragus and on the mastoid process, and note any discomfort or pain, suggesting otitis or mastoiditis. Some pain may be associated with toothache, a cold, a sore throat, or cervical spine injury. Inspect the ear canal for discharge (pus, mucus, blood, or cerebral spinal fluid [CSF]) and inflammation. Trauma can account for blood, mucus, and CSF in the ear canal. Check hearing acuity by covering one ear and whispering; then speaking into the other. Hearing loss may be accounted for by trauma, accumulation of debris (often cerumen), tympanic membrane rupture, drug use, and prolonged exposure to loud noise. Visualize the inner canal with the otoscope. With the largest speculum that will fit the canal, turn the patient's head away from you, pull the auricle slightly up and backward, and insert the otoscope. Inspect for wax (cerumen), discharge, redness, lesions, perforations, and foreign bodies. Then focus on the tympanic membrane. It should be a translucent pearly, white-to-pinkish gray. Color changes suggest fluid behind the eardrum, scarring, or infection. Also check for bulging, protractions, or perforations.

Visualize the patient's nose from the front and sides to determine any asymmetry, deviation, tenderness, flaring, or abnormal color. Tilt your patient's head back slightly and examine the nostrils. Insert the otoscope and check for deviation of the septum and perforations. Examine the nasal mucosa for color and the color, consistency, and quantity of drainage. Rhinitis (a runny nose) suggests seasonal allergies; a thick yellow discharge, infection; and blood, epistaxis from trauma or a septal defect. Test each side of the nose for patency by occluding the other side during a breath. There is normally some difference in patency between the sides. Palpate the frontal sinuses for swelling and tenderness.

Begin assessment of the mouth by observing the lips for color and condition. They should be pink, smooth, and symmetrical, without lesions, swelling, lumps, cracks, or scaliness. Using a bright light and tongue blade, examine the oral mucosa for color, lesions, white patches, or fissures. The mucosa should be pinkish red, smooth, and moist. The gums should be pink, with clearly defined margins around the teeth. The teeth should be well formed and straight. If the gums are swollen, bleed easily, and are separated from the teeth, suspect periodontal disease. Ask the patient to stick his tongue out and note its velvety surface. Hold the tongue with a 2 × 2 inch gauze pad and inspect all sides and the bottom. All surfaces should be pink and smooth. Then examine the pharynx and have the patient say "aaaahhh" while you hold the tongue down with a tongue blade. Watch the movement of the uvula and the coloration and condition of the palatine tonsils and posterior pharynx. Look for any pus, swelling, ulcers, or drainage. Also notice any odors, including alcohol, feces (bowel obstruction), acetone (diabetic ketoacidosis), gastric contents, coffee-grounds–like material (gastric hemorrhage), pink-tinged sputum (pulmonary edema), or bitter almonds (cyanide poisoning).

Neck   **pp. 82–84**

Inspect your patient's neck for symmetry and visible masses. Note any deformity, deviations, tugging, scars, gland enlargement, or visible lymph nodes. Examine for any open wounds and cover them with an occlusive dressing. Examine the jugular veins for distention while the patient is seated upright and at a 45° incline. Palpate the trachea to ensure it is in line. Palpate the thyroid while the patient swallows to ensure it is small, smooth, and without nodules. Palpate each lymph node to determine size, shape, tenderness, consistency, and mobility. Tender, swollen, and mobile nodes suggest inflammation from infection; hard and fixed ones suggest malignancy.

5. Describe the assessment of visual acuity.   **pp. 62–71**

Visual acuity is the ability to read detail. A wall chart with lines of progressively smaller letters is placed at 20 feet from the patient. He then reads to the smallest line in which he can recognize at least one-half the letters. The result is recorded as the distance from the chart and the distance at which a person with normal sight could distinguish the letters, 20/20 for normal or 20/60 for someone who reads what is normally read at 60 feet.

6. Explain the rationale for the use of an ophthalmoscope and otoscope.   pp. 37, 70–71, 75–78

The ophthalmoscope is a light source and a series of lenses that permit you to examine the interior of the patient's eyes. It allows you to examine the retina, blood vessels, and optic nerve at the back of the posterior chamber of the eye.

The otoscope is a light source and a magnifying lens that permit examination of a patient's ears and nose. The otoscope allows you to examine the external auditory canal and the tympanic membrane for trauma, irritation, or infection.

8. Describe percussion of the chest.   pp. 89, 91

Percuss both the anterior and posterior chest surfaces, examining for resonant (normal), hyperresonant (air-filled pneumothorax or tension pneumothorax), or dull sounds (fluid-filled hemothorax). Percuss both sides symmetrically from the apex to the base at 5-centimeter intervals, avoiding the scapulae. Determine the boundaries of any hyperresonance or dullness.

9. Differentiate the percussion notes and their characteristics.   pp. 33–34

Percussion provides three basic sounds: dull, resonant, and hyperresonant. Dull reflects a density and is a medium-pitched thud. It is usually caused by a dense organ (such as the liver) or fluid (such as blood) underneath. Resonant sounds are generally associated with a less dense tissue, such as the lungs, and are lower-pitched and longer-lasting sounds. Hyperresonant sounds reflect air, or air under pressure, and are the lowest-pitched sounds and the ones that diminish in volume most slowly.

The following objectives, although not listed in the chapter, will help in your understanding of the chapter content.

*Identify and describe the vital signs.   pp. 40–48

Pulse is the wave of pressure generated by the heart as it expels blood into the arterial system. It is measured by palpating a distal artery (or auscultated during blood pressure determination) and is evaluated for rate, rhythm, and quality (strength). The normal pulse is strong and regular, with a rate of 60 to 80 beats per minute.

Respiration is the movement of air through the airway and into and out of the lungs. It is evaluated by observing and/or feeling chest excursion and listening to air movement. The rate, effort, and quality (depth and pattern) of respirations are determined. Normal respiration moves a tidal volume of 500 mL at a rate of 12 to 20 times per minute with symmetrical chest wall movement.

Blood pressure is the force of blood against the arterial wall during the cardiac/pulse cycle. It is measured using a sphygmomanometer (blood pressure cuff) and stethoscope. The maximum, or systolic, blood pressure (the reading obtained when the ventricles contract); the lower, or diastolic, blood pressure (the reading obtained when the ventricles relax); and the difference between them (the pulse pressure) are evaluated. The systolic pressure is usually between 100 and 135 and the diastolic between 60 and 80.

Temperature is the body core temperature and is the product of heat-creating metabolism and body heat loss. It is measured by a glass or an electronic thermometer placed in the axilla, mouth, or rectum. Normal body temperature is 98.6°F (37°C).

*Identify and explain the importance of additional assessment techniques.   pp. 48–51

Pulse oximetry is the noninvasive measurement of oxygen saturation in the tissue of a distal extremity. It provides a real-time evaluation of oxygen delivery to the distal circulation. Normal readings are between 96 and 100 percent. Readings below this reflect problems with either respiration or circulation and demand intervention.

Capnography is the real-time evaluation of CO_2 in exhaled air. There are two types of end-tidal CO_2 monitors: small, disposable colormetric devices that change color in the presence of carbon dioxide and electronic devices that provide either a light indicating a minimum CO_2 content or a digital or wave-form display giving the concentration. Both devices are used to confirm proper endotracheal tube placement.

©2009 Pearson Education, Inc.
Paramedic Care: Principles & Practice, Vol. 2, 3rd. Ed.

Cardiac monitoring uses electronics to display the electrical activity of the heart. The monitor shows an electronic or paper tracing of the heart's activity—a normal rhythm, a dysrhythmia, or no activity (asystole). This information is essential to identifying when to shock the heart back to a normal rhythm or to treat it through the use of medication.

Blood glucose determination is performed by using a glucometer, a small electronic device that evaluates the color of a blood-stained reagent strip. The glucose level can rule out or identify hypoglycemia in a patient with a lowered level of consciousness or in a known diabetic.

Case Study Review

Reread the case study on pages 28 and 29 in Paramedic Care: Patient Assessment *before reading the following discussion.*

This case study clearly shows the benefit of a planned and well-directed physical examination of a patient with nonspecific signs and symptoms of disease. Here, Dale and Pam use the assessment to search out the possible causes, then converge, through specific signs and symptoms, on the patient's problem, which is their field diagnosis.

Dale and Pam arrive to care for a patient with very confusing and nonspecific signs and symptoms of illness. They and their patient, Mr. Dalton, count heavily on the comprehensive physical assessment to help sort out what might be wrong. A case like this is one of the few times you, as a paramedic, will employ most of the elements of a complete and detailed physical exam. More frequently, you will quickly identify the likely causes of your patient's chief complaint and presenting signs and symptoms—a differential diagnosis. Then you will focus your assessment on evaluating the presenting signs and symptoms and looking for those commonly associated with the diseases you suspect. This information then helps you rule out or support a problem, arriving at a single suspected problem—the field diagnosis.

Dale and Pam perform a quick primary survey to evaluate Mr. Dalton's mental status and ABCs. His first few words demonstrate that he is conscious and alert, and his airway and breathing are more than adequate. His mental status suggests his brain is being well perfused, and a quick pulse check confirms good circulation. With the elements of the primary survey complete, Dale and Pam move to the focused history and physical exam without a clear idea of what might be affecting Mr. Dalton.

Mr. Dalton's presentation is nonspecific to a particular medical problem; therefore, they must use the focused history and physical exam to investigate his physical and mental state more carefully. Elements of the patient history begin to direct their investigation toward a vascular problem: a history of coronary artery disease, hypertension, and the use of certain medications—nitroglycerin, aspirin, and digoxin. (Through his training and experience, Dale knows that nitroglycerin is given to reduce the demands on a heart with limited perfusion, that aspirin is used to reduce the risk of clot development, and that digoxin is often given for atrial fibrillation, which is frequently associated with pulmonary and cerebral emboli.) Added to the physical assessment finding—general weakness and an unstable walk and stance—what Dale and Pam learn suggests a motor or neurologic problem.

The team takes a quick set of vital signs that reveal only an abnormally high blood pressure, which is consistent with the history of hypertension. Dale performs the elements of the general survey and examines Mr. Dalton's appearance, level of consciousness, signs of distress, state of health, vital statistics, sexual development, skin color and lesions, posture, gait and motor activity, dress, grooming and personal hygiene, body or breath odor, and facial expression. They reveal a patient in generally good health with an appropriate affect. The only noted problem is one of coordinated walking (gait). The detailed physical exam reflects spasms at the outer reaches of left lateral eye movement, termed nystagmus. This, coupled with the gait problem, suggests a neurologic problem, for which Dale begins a complete neurologic exam.

Dale investigates posture, balance, reflexes, and coordination. Clearly, Mr. Dalton is slumped to the left side. Dale finds balance problems with Mr. Dalton, who drifts to the left when his eyes are closed. His reflexes are normal, at least for a 70-year-old man. His complaint about buttoning his shirt suggests a coordination problem, which Dale investigates further. He employs a few repetitive action exercises (thumb touch, shin touch, and palm-up/palm-down to thigh), which reveal a clear neurologic deficit on Mr. Dalton's left side.

Because of the left-sided slumping, nystagmus, and impaired coordination, Dale concludes that this is a cerebellar problem, most likely resulting from an arterial blockage. This is supported by both the history of earlier, less significant events (possibly transient ischemic events and an evolving stroke) and the vascular disease history discovered earlier. Note that motor and sensory function are controlled by the contralateral side of the brain (cerebral injury) and coordination is controlled by the ipsilateral cerebellum. In this scenario, Dale and Pam would also be likely to apply the cardiac monitor and evaluate the ECG for dysrhythmia. They might also auscultate the carotid arteries for bruit, suggestive of vascular disease that may be the origin of an embolus. In some EMS systems, stroke patients may be given clot-busting drugs, such as TPA or streptokinase, to dissolve blockage and reduce the effects of the infarct. In such a system, Dale and Pam may have a series of questions to ask of Mr. Dalton, to rule out the risk of internal hemorrhage, to help specifically identify the type of stroke or cerebrovascular accident, and to reduce the time from infarct to medication.

Content Self-Evaluation

MULTIPLE CHOICE

_____ 1. Of the physical examination techniques used in prehospital care, which is the least invasive?
- A. inspection
- B. auscultation
- C. palpation
- D. percussion
- E. C and D

_____ 2. "Crackles" would be found using which of the following assessment techniques?
- A. palpation
- B. auscultation
- C. inspection
- D. percussion
- E. none of the above

_____ 3. "Tenderness" would be discovered using which of the following assessment techniques?
- A. palpation
- B. auscultation
- C. inspection
- D. percussion
- E. none of the above

_____ 4. Which of the following techniques should be performed first during the physical examination?
- A. palpation
- B. auscultation
- C. inspection
- D. percussion
- E. none of the above

_____ 5. Which part of the hands and fingers is best suited to evaluate tissue consistency?
- A. tips of the fingers
- B. pads of the fingers
- C. palm of the hand
- D. back of the hands or fingers
- E. none of the above

_____ 6. Which part of the hands and fingers is best suited to evaluate vibration?
- A. tips of the fingers
- B. pads of the fingers
- C. palm of the hand
- D. back of the hands or fingers
- E. none of the above

_____ 7. Noticing areas of warmth during palpation might reflect an injury before significant edema and discoloration develop.
- A. True
- B. False

_____ 8. The booming sound produced by percussing an air-filled region is:
- A. hyperresonance.
- B. dull.
- C. resonance.
- D. flat.
- E. none of the above.

©2009 Pearson Education, Inc.
Paramedic Care: Principles & Practice, Vol. 2, 3rd. Ed.

_____ 9. The only region where you perform auscultation as other than the last step of assessment is the:
   A. anterior thorax.
   B. neck.
   C. abdomen.
   D. peripheral arteries.
   E. posterior thorax.

_____ 10. A heart rate above 100 beats per minute is known as:
   A. bradycardia.
   B. tachycardia.
   C. hypercardia.
   D. tachypnea.
   E. bradypnea.

_____ 11. One likely cause of bradycardia is:
   A. fever.
   B. pain.
   C. parasympathetic stimulation.
   D. fear.
   E. blood loss.

_____ 12. Which of the following is NOT an aspect of pulse evaluation?
   A. volume
   B. rhythm
   C. quality
   D. rate
   E. none of the above

_____ 13. Normal exhalation is:
   A. an active process involving accessory muscles.
   B. an active process involving the diaphragm and intercostal muscles.
   C. active in its early stages and passive in later stages.
   D. passive in its early stages and active in later stages.
   E. a passive process.

_____ 14. For a patient with an airway obstruction, exhalation is likely to be:
   A. an active process involving accessory muscles.
   B. an active process involving only the diaphragm and intercostal muscles.
   C. active in its early stages and passive in later stages.
   D. passive in its early stages and active in later stages.
   E. a passive process.

_____ 15. The amount of air a patient moves into and out of his lungs in one breath is the:
   A. normal volume.
   B. respiratory volume.
   C. residual volume.
   D. tidal volume.
   E. minute volume.

_____ 16. The pressure of the blood within the blood vessels while the ventricles are relaxing is the:
   A. Korotkoff blood pressure.
   B. systolic blood pressure.
   C. diastolic blood pressure.
   D. asystolic blood pressure.
   E. atrial blood pressure.

_____ 17. The diastolic blood pressure represents a measure of:
   A. systemic vascular resistance.
   B. the cardiac output.
   C. the viscosity of the blood.
   D. the strength of ventricular contraction.
   E. relative blood volume.

_____ 18. Which of the following could influence a patient's blood pressure?
   A. anxiety
   B. position (lying, sitting, standing)
   C. recent smoking
   D. eating
   E. all of the above

_____ 19. Generally, hypertension in a healthy adult is any blood pressure higher than:
   A. 120/80.
   B. 140/90.
   C. 160/90.
   D. 180/100.
   E. 200/100.

_____ 20. What is the pulse pressure in a patient with the following vital signs: pulse 82 and strong; respirations 14 and full; and blood pressure 144/96?
A. 14
B. 40
C. 48
D. 96
E. 120

_____ 21. In the tilt test, what vital sign change is a positive sign of hypovolemia?
A. Blood pressure drops by 10 to 20 mmHg.
B. Blood pressure rises by 10 to 20 mmHg.
C. Pulse rate drops by 10 to 20 beats per minute.
D. Pulse rate rises by 10 to 20 beats per minute.
E. Either A or D is correct.

_____ 22. Hyperthermia can result from all of the following EXCEPT:
A. high environmental temperatures.
B. infections.
C. reduced metabolic activity.
D. drugs.
E. increases in metabolic activity.

_____ 23. What technique of stethoscope use best transmits low-pitched sound to the ear?
A. light pressure on the diaphragm
B. firm pressure on the diaphragm
C. moderate pressure on the bell
D. light pressure on the bell
E. strong pressure on the bell

_____ 24. The bell of a stethoscope is best for listening to the sounds of:
A. blood vessel bruits.
B. the blood pressure.
C. the heart.
D. the lung.
E. none of the above.

_____ 25. Which of the following is NOT a characteristic of a good stethoscope?
A. thick, heavy tubing
B. long tubing (70 to 100 cm)
C. snug-fitting earpieces
D. a bell with a rubber-ring edge
E. all of the above

_____ 26. Generally, each narrow line on a sphygmomanometer represents what pressure difference?
A. 1 mmHg
B. 2 mmHg
C. 4 mmHg
D. 5 mmHg
E. 10 mmHg

_____ 27. If a patient has a regular and strong pulse, you should determine the pulse rate by assessing the number of beats in:
A. 2 minutes and dividing by 2.
B. 3 minutes.
C. 30 seconds and multiplying by 2.
D. 15 seconds and multiplying by 4.
E. 10 seconds and multiplying by 5.

_____ 28. Use of which of the following pulse points is recommended with a small child?
A. radial
B. brachial
C. carotid
D. popliteal
E. dorsalis pedis

_____ 29. It is important to attempt to evaluate your patient's respiratory rate and volume without his being aware of it.
A. True
B. False

_____ 30. The proper position of the patient's arm when taking the blood pressure is:
A. arm slightly flexed.
B. palm up.
C. fingers relaxed.
D. clothing removed from the upper arm.
E. all of the above.

©2009 Pearson Education, Inc.
Paramedic Care: Principles & Practice, Vol. 2, 3rd. Ed.

_____ 31. The sphygmomanometer should be inflated to what level beyond the point at which the patient's radial pulse disappears?
A. 10 mmHg
B. 20 mmHg
C. 30 mmHg
D. 40 mmHg
E. between B and C

_____ 32. The first blood pressure reading is the systolic blood pressure, indicated by the early deflections of the sphygmomanometer needle.
A. True
B. False

_____ 33. When using an oral glass thermometer, it should be left in the mouth for what period of time?
A. 30 to 45 seconds
B. 30 to 60 seconds
C. 1 to 2 minutes
D. 2 minutes
E. 3 to 4 minutes

_____ 34. The normal patient oxygen saturation without supplemental oxygen at sea level should be:
A. 90 to 95 percent.
B. below 95 percent.
C. 100 percent.
D. 96 to 100 percent.
E. below 90 percent.

_____ 35. A patient suffering from carbon monoxide poisoning will likely have a pulse oximetry reading that is:
A. accurate.
B. falsely high.
C. falsely low.
D. erratic and inaccurate.
E. unreadable.

_____ 36. The ECG of a cardiac monitor can tell you all of the following EXCEPT:
A. the heart rate.
B. the sequence of cardiac events.
C. the timing of cardiac events.
D. the pumping ability of the heart.
E. both A and C.

_____ 37. The skin regulates body temperature through:
A. radiation.
B. evaporation.
C. conduction.
D. convection.
E. all of the above.

_____ 38. Pale skin is least likely to be caused by which of the following?
A. increased deoxyhemoglobin
B. a cold environment
C. shock compensation
D. anemia
E. hypovolemic shock

_____ 39. Which of the following skin discolorations represents a yellow hue?
A. cyanosis
B. jaundice
C. eccyhmosis
D. erythema
E. pallor

_____ 40. A heavy scaling of the skin under the hair is:
A. dandruff.
B. nits.
C. seborrheic dermatitis.
D. psoriasis.
E. none of the above.

_____ 41. With age, the toenails are likely to become:
A. hard.
B. thick.
C. brittle.
D. yellowish.
E. all of the above.

_____ 42. The bluish discoloration around the orbits of the eyes, suggestive of a basilar skull fracture, is called:
A. racoon eyes.
B. Battle's sign.
C. periorbital ecchymosis.
D. retroauricular ecchymosis.
E. either A or C.

_____ 43. The cranial nerves that control eye movement are:
   A. I, II, and III.   D. II, VI, and VII.
   B. II, III, and IV.   E. V, VI, and VIII.
   C. III, IV, and VI.

_____ 44. The muscular and colored portion of the eye that constricts and dilates to regulate
   light falling on the retinal surface is the:
   A. retina.   D. iris.
   B. pupil.   E. lens.
   C. conjunctiva.

_____ 45. The characteristic of the unaffected eye responding to stimuli in the affected
   eye is:
   A. consensual response.   D. ipsilateral response.
   B. direct response.   E. none of the above.
   C. simultaneous response.

_____ 46. About 20 percent of the population have a noticeable difference in the size
   of the pupils, a condition called:
   A. hyphema.   D. hypopyon.
   B. anisocoria.   E. none of the above.
   C. glaucoma.

_____ 47. The ear provides what important body function beyond hearing?
   A. equalization of pressure during yawning
   B. vibration sensation
   C. balance and head position sense
   D. equalization of body and outside pressure
   E. all of the above except B

_____ 48. Otorrhea is a discharge from the ear that may contain:
   A. pus.   D. cerebrospinal fluid.
   B. mucus.   E. all of the above.
   C. blood.

_____ 49. The term for a common nosebleed is:
   A. epistaxis.   D. rhinitis.
   B. otorrhea.   E. none of the above.
   C. rhinorrhea.

_____ 50. The most superior and prominent airway structure in the neck is the:
   A. cricoid cartilage.   D. thyroid gland.
   B. thyroid cartilage.   E. jugular vein.
   C. tracheal ring.

Special Project

Vital Signs

For each of the following vital signs, list the normal range of values and any other important consider-ations in their evaluation.

Pulse:

_____

_____

_____

©2009 Pearson Education, Inc.
Paramedic Care: Principles & Practice, Vol. 2, 3rd. Ed.

Respirations:

_____

_____

_____

_____

_____

_____

Blood pressure:

_____

_____

_____

_____

_____

_____

Temperature:

_____

_____

_____

_____

_____

_____

_____

Section II, pp. 84–136

Review of Chapter Objectives

After reading this chapter, you should be able to:

4. Describe the examination of the following body regions, differentiate between normal and abnormal findings, and define the significance of abnormal findings.

Thorax (anterior and posterior)   pp. 84–92

To assess the chest, you need a stethoscope with a bell and diaphragm. Expose the entire thorax with consideration for the patient's dignity and modesty and inspect, palpate, percuss, and auscultate. Compare findings from one side of the chest to those from the other and from posterior to anterior. Look for general shape and symmetry as well as for the rate and pattern of breathing. Observe for retractions and the use of accessory muscles (suggestive of airway obstruction or restriction) and palpate for deformities, tenderness, crepitus (suggestive of rib fracture), and abnormal chest excursion (suggestive of flail chest or spinal injury). Feel for vibrations associated with air movement and speech. Percuss the chest for dullness (hemothorax, pleural effusion, or pneumonia), resonance, and hyperresonance (pneumothorax or tension pneumothorax). Finally, auscultate the lung lobes for normal breath sounds, crackles (pulmonary edema), wheezes (asthma), rhonchi, stridor (airway obstruction), and pleural friction rubs.

Arterial pulse, including rate, rhythm, and amplitude pp. 92–97
Locate a soft and pulsing carotid artery in the neck, just lateral to the cricoid cartilage to avoid pressure on the carotid sinus. Carefully press down until the pulse wave just lifts your finger off the artery. Determine the rate and carefully evaluate for regularity. Irregularity may be caused by dysrhythmia, while variation in strength may be due to such phenomena as pulsus paradoxus, increasing strength with exhalation and decreasing with inhalation. Also note any thrills (humming or vibration) and listen with the stethoscope for bruits (sounds of turbulent flow).

Jugular venous pressure and pulsations pp. 92–97
Examine the anterior neck and locate the jugular veins. Position your patient with his head elevated 30° and turned away from you. Look for pulsation just above the suprasternal notch. Identify the highest point of pulsation and measure the distance from the sternal angle. The highest point of pulsation is usually between 1 and 2 cm from the sternal angle. (Distention when the patient is elevated at higher angles may reflect tension pneumothorax or pericardial tamponade, whereas flat veins at lower angles may suggest hypovolemia.)

Abdomen pp. 92–97
Question your patient regarding any pain, tenderness, or unusual feeling, as well as recent bowel and bladder function. Carefully inspect the area for scars, dilated veins, stretch marks, rashes, lesions, and pigmentation changes. Discoloration around the umbilicus (Cullen's sign) or over the flanks (Grey Turner's sign) suggests intra-abdominal hemorrhage. Assess the size and shape of the abdomen, determining whether it is scaphoid (concave), flat, round, or distended, and look for any bulges or hernias. Ascites results in bulges in the flanks and across the abdomen, suggesting congestive heart or liver failure, while suprapubic bulges suggest a full bladder or pregnant uterus. Look also for any masses, palpations, or peristalsis. A slight vascular pulsing is normal, but excessive movement suggests an aneurysm. Auscultate and percuss as described earlier. Then depress each quadrant gently and release. Look for patient expression or muscle guarding suggestive of injury or peritonitis.

Male and female genitalia pp. 103–107
Ensure patient privacy, a warm environment, and patient modesty during the exam; also be sure the patient has emptied his bladder before beginning. Expose only those body areas that you must, and explain what you are going to do before you do it. Inspect the genitalia for development and maturity. Visually inspect the mons pubis, labia, and perineum of the female patient for swelling, lesions, or irritation suggestive of a sebaceous cyst or sexually transmitted disease. Check the hair bases for small, red maculopapules suggestive of lice. Retract the labia and inspect the inner labia and urethral opening. Examine for a white, curdy discharge (fungal infection) or yellow-green discharge (bacterial infection). For the male, inspect the penis and testicles, noting inflammation and lesions suggestive of sexually transmitted disease. Check for lice and examine the glans for degeneration, inflammation, or discharge. Yellow discharge is reflective of gonorrhea.

Anus and rectum pp. 107–108
Position your patient on his left side with legs flexed and buttocks near the edge of the stretcher. Be sensitive to the patient's feelings and drape or cover any areas not being observed. With a gloved hand, spread the buttocks apart and examine the area for lumps, ulcers, inflammations, rashes, or lesions. Palpate any areas carefully, noting inflammation or tenderness. If appropriate, obtain a fecal sample for testing.

Musculoskeletal system pp. 108–138
Advancing age causes changes in the musculoskeletal system, including shortening and increased curvature of the spine, a reduction in muscle mass and strength, and a reduction in the range of motion. Observe the patient's general posture, build, and muscular development as well as the movement of the extremities, gait, and position at rest. Then inspect all regions of the body for deformities, symmetry and symmetrical movement, joint structure, and swelling, nodules, or

©2009 Pearson Education, Inc.
Paramedic Care: Principles & Practice, Vol. 2, 3rd. Ed.

inflammation. Deformities are often related to misaligned articulating bones, dislocations, or subluxations. Impaired movement is usually related to arthritis; nodules are related to rheumatic fever or rheumatoid arthritis; and redness is related to gout, rheumatic fever, or arthritis. Compare dissimilar joints to determine what structures might be affected. Assess range of motion by moving the limb, ask the patient to move the limb, and then ask the patient to move the limb against resistance. Note any asymmetry and inequality between active and passive motion. Also examine for crepitation (a grating vibration or sound) that may suggest arthritis, an inflamed joint, or a fracture. Avoid manipulating a deformed or painful joint. Perform a physical exam on each joint, moving it through its normal range of motion and noting any deformities, limited or resistant movement, tenderness, and swelling.

7. Describe the survey of respiration. pp. 84–92

The survey of the chest assesses the thorax and respiration by inspection, palpation, percussion, and auscultation. Compare findings side to side and anterior to back. Visualize and auscultate the five lung lobes during your exam. Examine the patient's respiration, looking for increased inspiratory or expiratory time or any sounds indicating upper or lower airway obstruction. Examine the chest for symmetry and symmetry of motion and any retraction or any anterior-posterior dimension abnormality. Also feel for any unusual vibrations associated with speech. Percuss the chest and note any hyperresonance or dullness. Listen through the stethoscope for lung sounds over each lobe and note any crackles or wheezes. Identify the respiratory rate and volume of each breath and determine the minute volume.

10. Describe special examination techniques related to the assessment of the chest. pp. 84–92

Chest excursion
Place your hands at the 10th intercostal space with the fingers spread and feel for chest excursion as the patient breathes deeply. Your hand should move equally about 3 to 5 cm with each breath.

Fremitus
Place a cupped hand against the chest wall at various locations and feel for vibrations while the patient says "ninety-nine" or "one-on-one." These vibrations should be equal throughout the chest. Note any enhanced, decreased, or absent fremitus.

Diaphragm excursion
Percuss the border of the rib cage for the dullness of the diaphragm during quiet breathing. Then mark the highest and lowest movement during respiration. Repeat the process on the other side of the chest. This excursion should be about 6 cm and equal on each side.

11. Describe the auscultation of the chest, heart, and abdomen.

Chest pp. 88–92
Have your patient breathe more deeply and slowly than normal with an open mouth. Using the stethoscope's disk, auscultate each side of the chest from the apex to the base every 5 cm, listening at each location for one full breath.

Heart pp. 93–97
Using the diaphragm of the stethoscope, listen for heart sounds at the 2nd through 5th intercostal spaces at both sternal borders and at the point of maximum impulse (PMI). Repeat the process using the bell of the stethoscope to discern lower-pitched sounds.

Abdomen pp. 101–103
Using the stethoscope's disk, auscultate each abdominal quadrant for at least 30 seconds to 1 minute.

12. Distinguish between normal and abnormal auscultation findings of the chest, heart, and abdomen and explain their significance.

Chest pp. 88–92
Normal breath sounds are the quiet sounds (almost low-pitched sighs) of air moving. Abnormal breath sounds are termed "adventitious" and include the following. Any crackles

(a light crackling, popping, nonmusical sound) suggest fluid in the smaller airways. Late inspiratory crackles suggest heart failure or interstitial lung disease, whereas early crackles suggest heart failure or chronic bronchitis. Wheezes (more musical notes) denote obstruction of the smaller airways. The closer they appear to inspiration, the more serious is the obstruction. Stridor is a high-pitched, loud inspiratory wheeze reflective of laryngeal or tracheal obstruction. Grating or squeaking sounds describe pleural friction rubs and occur as the pleural layers become inflamed, then rub together. You may also listen for sound transmission while the patient speaks. Bronchophony occurs when you hear the words "ninety-nine" abnormally clearly through the stethoscope, a suggestion that blood, fluid, or a tumor has replaced normal tissue. Assess for whispered pectoriloquy by asking the patient to whisper "ninety-nine"; unusually clear sounds indicate an abnormal condition. Egophony occurs when you can hear the sound of long "e" as "a" when vocal resonance is abnormally increased.

Heart   pp. 93–97
The normal heart produces a "lub-dub" sound heard through the disk of the stethoscope with each cardiac contraction. The "lub" and "dub" may split when valves close out of sync, "la-lub-dub" reflects an S1 split; "lub-da-dub" is an S2 split. S2 splitting is normal in children and young adults, though abnormal in older adults if expiratory or persistent splitting occurs. S3 splitting produces a "lub-dub-dee" cadence, such as the word "Kentucky." It occurs commonly in children and young adults but reflects blood filling a dilated ventricle and may suggest ventricular failure in the patient over 30. The S4 heart sound is the "dee" sound of "dee-lub-dub" with a cadence similar to the word "Tennessee." It develops from vibrations as the atrium pushes blood into a ventricle that resists filling, suggestive of heart failure.

Abdomen   pp. 101–103
Normal bowel sounds consist of a variety of high-pitched gurgles and clicks that occur every 5 to 15 seconds. More frequent activity suggests an increase in bowel motility, and especially loud and prolonged gurgling sounds (borborygmi) indicate hyperperistalsis. Decreased or absent sounds suggest a paralytic ileus or peritonitis. You may also hear swishing sounds (bruit) over the major vessels, suggesting a vascular defect, such as aneurysm or stenosis.

13. **Describe special techniques of the cardiovascular examination.**   pp. 92–97

Inspection for signs of cardiovascular insufficiency
Examine the extremities for signs of insufficiency, including pallor, delayed capillary refill, temperature variation, and dependent edema. Then assess the carotid arteries for pulse strength, rate, and rhythm. Does the rate or strength vary with respirations? Do you feel thrills (feel a humming sensation)? If so, auscultate for bruits.

Jugular vein distention
Position the patient supine with the head elevated 30° and turned away from the side being assessed. Look for pulsations of the external jugular vein on either side of the trachea just before it passes behind the manubrium. Locate the highest point of pulsation and measure the distance from the sternal angle. Normal venous pressure distends the vein above the clavicle between 1 and 2 cm. Examine both jugulars for symmetrical pulsing and distention.

Point of Maximum Impulse (PMI)
Have the patient lie comfortably with his head elevated 30°. Inspect and palpate the chest for the apical impulse, or the PMI. It is normally at the 5th intercostal space, midclavicular line. In muscular or obese patients, you may need to percuss the point (dull vs. resonant).

©2009 Pearson Education, Inc.
Paramedic Care: Principles & Practice, Vol. 2, 3rd. Ed.

Content Self-Evaluation

MULTIPLE CHOICE

_____ 1. The layer of tissue that covers the interior of the chest wall and helps ensure that the lungs move with the thorax is the:
A. visceral pleura.
B. parietal pleura.
C. pertioneum.
D. pulmonary pleura.
E. perineum.

_____ 2. A likely location to notice retraction during forced inspiration is:
A. the suprasternal notch.
B. the intercostal spaces.
C. the supraclavicular space.
D. all of the above.
E. none of the above.

_____ 3. The type of motion associated with a free segment of the chest where the segment moves opposite to the rest of the chest during breathing is:
A. symbiotic.
B. paradoxical.
C. antagonistic.
D. retractive.
E. traumatic.

_____ 4. During the palpation of the chest, you should feel for which of the following?
A. tenderness
B. deformities
C. depressions
D. asymmetry
E. all of the above

_____ 5. During the check for chest excursion, the distance between your thumbs should increase by what amount during the patient's inspiration?
A. 2 cm
B. 3 to 5 cm
C. 5 to 6 cm
D. 10 to 12 cm
E. 0 cm

_____ 6. Increased tactile fremitus suggests which of the following conditions?
A. pneumonia
B. pneumothorax
C. pleural effusion
D. emphysema
E. all of the above

_____ 7. Which condition is most likely to cause an area of the lung that is dull to percussion?
A. pneumothorax
B. tension pneumothorax
C. hemothorax
D. pericardial tamponade
E. friction rubs

_____ 8. Light popping, nonmusical sounds heard in the chest during inspiration are known as:
A. rhonchi.
B. stridor.
C. crackles.
D. wheezes.
E. none of the above.

_____ 9. Hearing words transmitted clearly as you auscultate the chest with the stethoscope is a normal finding called bronchophony.
A. True
B. False

_____ 10. The point of maximal impulse (PMI) in the adult is usually located at the:
A. 3rd costal cartilage, close to the sternum.
B. 3rd intercostal space, just left of the sternum.
C. 5th intercostal space, just right of the sternum.
D. 5th intercostal space, near the midclavicular line.
E. 8th intercostal space, near the midclavicular line.

11. Which listing represents the valves of the heart in order as blood flows through them from the vena cavae?
   A. tricuspid, pulmonic, mitral, aortic
   B. mitral, aortic, tricuspid, pulmonic
   C. pulmonic, tricuspid, aortic, mitral
   D. aortic, tricuspid, pulmonic, mitral
   E. tricuspid, aortic, mitral, pulmonic

12. The "lub" of the heart sounds represents which event of the cardiac cycle?
   A. ejection of blood from the ventricles
   B. ventricular contraction
   C. ventricular filling
   D. closing of the aortic and pulmonic valves
   E. closing of the tricuspid and mitral valves

13. Which of the following elements does NOT affect cardiac output?
   A. heart rate
   B. cardiac preload
   C. contractile force
   D. hematocrit
   E. peripheral vascular resistance

14. Which of the following does NOT inhibit venous return to the heart?
   A. peripheral vascular resistance
   B. hypovolemia
   C. tension pneumothorax
   D. cardiac tamponade
   E. congestive heart failure

15. Which abdominal organ is found in all four quadrants?
   A. stomach
   B. liver
   C. large intestine
   D. pancreas
   E. spleen

16. An eccyhmotic discoloration over the umbilicus is:
   A. Grey Turner's sign.
   B. borborygmi.
   C. Hering-Breuer sign.
   D. Cullen's sign.
   E. none of the above.

17. Auscultation of high-pitched gurgles and clicks every 5 to 15 seconds in the abdomen indicates:
   A. borborygmi.
   B. increased bowel motility.
   C. absent bowel sounds.
   D. normal bowel sounds.
   E. ascites.

18. The fleshy folds that cover the vagina are the:
   A. labia.
   B. clitoris.
   C. mons pubis.
   D. perineum.
   E. menarche.

19. The sound or feeling caused by unlubricated bone ends rubbing together is:
   A. palpable fremitus.
   B. crepitation.
   C. bruit.
   D. friction rub.
   E. the pooh-pooh sign.

20. The type of movement permitted between the phalanges is:
   A. abduction/adduction.
   B. rotation.
   C. flexion/extension.
   D. supination/pronation.
   E. both C and D.

21. Carpal tunnel syndrome involves which nerve?
   A. brachial
   B. median
   C. radial
   D. ulnar
   E. olecranon

©2009 Pearson Education, Inc.
Paramedic Care: Principles & Practice, Vol. 2, 3rd. Ed.

_____ 22. The type of movement permitted between the radius, ulna, and humerus is:
- A. abduction/adduction.
- B. rotation.
- C. flexion/extension.
- D. supination/pronation.
- E. both C and D.

_____ 23. The joint that has the greatest range of motion of any joint in the human body is the:
- A. shoulder.
- B. wrist.
- C. hip.
- D. elbow.
- E. ankle.

_____ 24. A major muscle of the calf is the:
- A. bicep.
- B. tricep.
- C. gastrocnemius.
- D. hamstring.
- E. gracilis anterior.

_____ 25. The knee joint involves all of the following bones EXCEPT the:
- A. femur.
- B. patella.
- C. tibia.
- D. fibula.
- E. all of the above.

_____ 26. The type of motion permitted by the knee joint is:
- A. flexion/extension.
- B. adduction/abduction.
- C. inversion/eversion.
- D. limited rotation.
- E. both A and D.

_____ 27. Which region of the spine is most mobile?
- A. cervical
- B. thoracic
- C. lumbar
- D. sacral
- E. coccygeal

_____ 28. The mid and lower cervical spine permits which type of movement?
- A. flexion
- B. extension
- C. lateral bending
- D. rotation
- E. all of the above

_____ 29. A lateral curvature of the spine is:
- A. lordosis.
- B. scoliosis.
- C. kyphosis.
- D. spina bifida.
- E. none of the above.

_____ 30. Tenderness at a vertebral process and in the surrounding musculature of the lumbar spine is most likely due to:
- A. vertebral process fracture.
- B. ligamentous injury.
- C. paravertebral muscular spasm.
- D. herniated intervertebral disk.
- E. none of the above.

Special Projects

Range of Motion Exercise

Identify the range of motion for each of the joints listed in the following chart as discussed in your reading. Then fill in the rest by reviewing the text, pages 11 through 129.

It is not easy to remember and evaluate the range of motion for each joint of the extremities. To help you both remember the ranges of motion for each joint and assess the mobility of the patients you will treat, test your own joints for their ranges of motion against those from the text (and the following chart). Identify the joints where your movement exceeds or is less than the figures given in the book. Remember this difference. Then if you ever question how a patient's range of movements relates to the normal ranges, compare the patient's joint mobility to your own.

Physical Assessment—Personal Benchmarking

To perform the physical assessment of a patient, you will need to use the skills of inspection, palpation, auscultation, and percussion. You must not only master each of these skills but also learn to recognize normal and abnormal patient presentations. Often the distinction between normal and abnormal is very small and difficult to recognize without extensive experience. It is also difficult to maintain the ability to differentiate between normal and abnormal signs unless you practice the skill regularly. To help in skills maintenance, frequently use yourself as a physiological model upon which to practice assessment techniques and as a benchmark against which you can measure your patients' responses.

Upper Extremity

Joint	Flexion/Extension	Rotation	Other Motion
Wrist	_____/_____		(Medial/Lateral) _____/_____
Elbow	_____/_____		(Supination/Pronation) _____/_____
Shoulder	_____/_____	(Internal/External) _____/_____	(Abduction/Adduction) _____/_____

Lower Extremity

Joint	Flexion/Extension	Rotation	Other Motion
Ankle	(Dorsiflex/Plantar Flex) _____/_____		(Inversion/Eversion) _____/_____
Knee	_____/_____		
Hip	_____/_____	(External/Internal) _____/_____	(Abduction) _____

Auscultation: You need a stethoscope for this exercise.

Apply the diaphragm of the stethoscope to the skin of your chest or abdomen. If you do not warm it first, you will be quite surprised at how cold it feels. Remember this as you are auscultating your patients' chests and abdomens.

Practice using the disk and diaphragm to ensure you know which setting sends bell sounds to your ears and which sends diaphragm sounds. Listen to the different sounds found at various locations around the chest and abdomen. Increase the pressure on the bell from gentle for low sounds to strong pressure for high-pitched sounds. You might also practice listening with the television on at various volume levels. This simulates background noise at the emergency scene and demonstrates how difficult it can be to assess breath, heart, and bowel sounds in the field.

Lung sounds: Review pages 84 through 92.

Listen to lung sounds in each of the five lung lobes. Remember that your patient's position will be reversed; his left lobes will be to your right. Take slow, deep breaths with your mouth open and listen

©2009 Pearson Education, Inc.
Paramedic Care: Principles & Practice, Vol. 2, 3rd. Ed.

for the faint noise of air moving through the small airways (normal or vesicular breath sounds). If you have a chance to auscultate your chest when you are experiencing the congestion of a cold, you may hear crackles or wheezes.

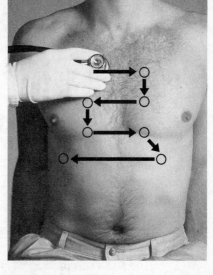

Then, auscultate the trachea at the suprasternal notch. Listen to the sounds; then move the diaphragm downward and laterally toward the lung fields. You will notice the quality of the sounds change as you move through the bronchial and bronchovesicular areas. Speak as you auscultate and notice how the speech sounds. It should be muffled, though you will hear it more clearly than when performing it on a patient, because some sound is transmitted through the bones of the face and skull in addition to the stethoscope.

Heart sounds: Review pages 92 through 97.

Review the accompanying illustration to identify the proper locations for auscultating the heart sounds. With each sound, increase the pressure on the bell from very light to heavy and appreciate the changing quality of the sounds. You might also palpate the carotid artery and then the radial pulse while auscultating to note the synchronization and delay between the sounds and pulse. Listen for the S1 and S2 sounds (the "lub-dub") of the normal heart.

Bowel sounds: Review pages 97 through 103.

Review the text on pages 101–103 and listen in each abdominal quadrant for at least 30 seconds to 1 minute with the diaphragm of your stethoscope. Listen very carefully in a very quiet environment because bowel sounds are difficult to decipher. Check your bowel sounds at various times during the day. They will likely be most frequent just before and right after a meal and before you go to sleep.

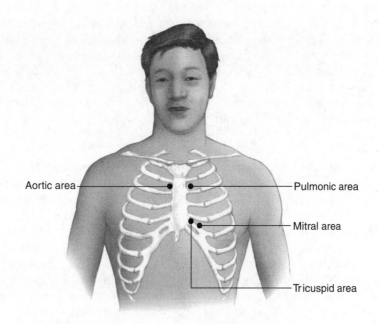

Aortic area — Pulmonic area

Mitral area

Tricuspid area

Review of Chapter Objectives

After reading this chapter, you should be able to:

2. Describe the evaluation of mental status. pp. 142–146

The evaluation of mental status begins with your interview. The evaluation permits you to determine your patient's level of responsiveness, general appearance, behavior, and speech. You specifically look at his appearance and behavior, speech and language skills, mood, thought and perception, insight and judgment, and memory and attention.

4. Describe the examination of the following body regions, differentiate between normal and abnormal findings, and define the significance of abnormal findings.

Heart and blood vessels pp. 136–142, 92–97

Examine the cardiovascular function by inspecting for skin pallor or other signs suggestive of arterial insufficiency or occlusion. Then evaluate carotid and peripheral pulses for rate, rhythm, and quality as well as the jugular vein for signs of distention (JVD). A heart rate above 100 is tachycardia and may be related to excitement and stress or shock, while a heart rate below 60 (bradycardia) may be related to an athlete's state of conditioning or head injury. Excessive JVD suggests right heart failure or cardiac tamponade, while abnormally low distention may suggest hypovolemia. Auscultate the heart sounds either side of the sternum at the 2nd intercostal space and the left side of the sternum at the 5th intercostal space. Variations of the normal "lub-dub" suggest cardiac abnormalities, though some variant sounds may be normal in children and young adults.

Peripheral vascular system pp. 136–142

Examine the upper, then the lower, extremities and compare them, one to another, for the following: size, symmetry, swelling, venous congestion, skin and nail bed color, temperature, skin texture, and turgor. Yellow and brittle nails, swollen digit ends (clubbing), or poor nail bed color suggests chronic arterial insufficiency. Assess the distal circulation, noting the strength, rate, and regularity of the pulse and comparing pulses bilaterally. If you have difficulty palpating a pulse or cannot find one, palpate a more proximal site. Feel the spongy compliance of the vessels, note their coloration, and examine for inflammation along the vein, indicative of deep vein thrombosis. Gently feel for edema and pitting edema in each distal extremity.

Nervous system pp. 142–167

To evaluate mental status and speech, examine your patient's appearance and behavior, speech and language, mood, thoughts and perceptions, and memory and attention. Observe the patient's appearance and behavior, level of consciousness, posture and motor behavior, appropriateness of dress, grooming and personal hygiene, and facial expression. Note any abnormal speech pattern and observe the patient's attitude toward you and others expressed both verbally and nonverbally. Note any excessive emotion or lack of emotion. Assess the patient's thoughts and perceptions. Are they realistic and socially acceptable? Question for any visions, voices, perceived odors, or feelings about things that are not there. Examine the patient's insights and judgments to determine if he knows what is happening. Assess the patient's memory and attention and determine his orientation to time, place, and person (sometimes considered as person and own person). Then test immediate, recent, and remote memory. Any deviation from a normal and expected response is to be noted and suggests illness or a psychiatric problem.

Begin the examination of the motor system by observing the patient for symmetry, deformities, and involuntary movements. Tremors or fasiculations while the patient is at rest suggest Parkinson's disease; their occurrence during motion suggests postural tremor. Determine muscle

©2009 Pearson Education, Inc.
Paramedic Care: Principles & Practice, Vol. 2, 3rd. Ed.

bulk, which is classified as normal, atrophy, hypertrophy, or pseudotrophy (bulk without strength, as in muscular dystrophy). Unilateral hand atrophy suggests median or ulnar nerve paralysis. Check tone by moving a relaxed limb through a range of motion. Describe any flaccidity or rigidity and then examine muscle strength, starting with grip strength and continuing through all limbs. Again note any asymmetry (the patient's dominant side should be slightly stronger). Observe the patient's gait and have him walk a straight line (heel to toe). Any ataxia suggests cerebellar disease, loss of position sense, or intoxication. Also have the patient walk on his toes, then heels; hop on each foot; and then do a shallow knee bend. Perform a Romberg test (have him stand with his feet together and eyes closed for 20 to 30 seconds). Any excessive sway (a positive Romberg test) suggests ataxia from loss of position sense, whereas an inability to maintain balance with eyes open represents cerebellar ataxia. Ask the patient to hold his arms straight out in front with his palms up and eyes closed. Pronation suggests mild hemiparesis; drifting sideways or upward suggests loss of positional sense. Ask your patient to perform various rapid, alternating movements and observe for smoothness, speed, and rhythm. The dominant side should perform best, and any slow, irregular, or clumsy movements suggest cerebellar or extrapyramidal disease. Have your patient touch his thumb rapidly with the tip of the index finger, place his hand on his thigh and rapidly alternate from palm up to down, and assess for point-to-point testing (touch his nose, then your index finger several times rapidly or, for the legs, have him touch heel to knee, then run it down the shin). Any jerking, difficulty in performing the task, or tremors suggest cerebellar disease. For position testing, have the patient perform the leg test with his eyes closed.

Evaluate the sensory system by testing sensations of pain, light touch, temperature, position, vibration, and discrimination. Compare responses bilaterally and from distal to proximal; then associate any deficit discovered with the dermatome it represents. Test superficial and deep tendon reflexes and note a dulled (cord or lower neuron damage) or hyperactive response (upper neuron disease).

Cranial nerves   pp. 146–154

CN-I is checked by evaluating the ability to sense odors in each nostril.

CN-II is checked by testing for visual acuity and field of view.

CN-III is checked by examining pupillary direct and consensual response.

CN-III, IV, and VI are checked by testing for smooth and unrestricted extraocular motion.

CN-V is checked by testing the masseter muscle strength and sensation on the forehead, cheek, chin, and cornea.

CN-VII is checked by examining the patient's face during conversations, looking for any asymmetry, eyelid droop, or abnormal movements.

CN-VIII is checked by evaluating for hearing and balance (with his eyes closed).

CN-IX and X are checked by evaluating speech, swallowing, saying "aaahhh," and the gag reflex.

CN-XI is checked by testing trapezius and sternocleidomastoid muscles at rest and by evaluating head turning and shoulder raising.

CN-XII is checked by evaluating speech and having the patient extend his tongue outward.

Any deviation from a normally expected response is a reason to suspect a cranial nerve injury.

14. Describe the general guidelines of recording examination information.   pp. 175–176

Use a standard format to organize the information. Use appropriate medical terminology and language. Present your findings legibly, accurately, and truthfully, remembering that your record will become a legal document. Include all data discovered in your assessment.

The standard organization for medical documentation is the S (Subjective), O (Objective), A (Assessment), and P (Plan) format (SOAP format):

Subjective information is what your patient or others tell you, including the chief complaint and the past and present medical history.

Objective information is that which you observe or determine during the scene size-up, primary survey, focused history and physical exam, detailed assessment, and ongoing assessments.

Assessment summarizes the findings to suggest a field diagnosis.

Plan is the further diagnosis, treatment, and patient education you intend to offer.

15. Discuss the examination considerations for an infant or child. pp. 167–174

Children are not small adults but patients with special physiological and psychological differences. In general, remain calm and confident, establish a rapport with the parents, and have them help with the exam. Provide positive feedback to both the child and the parents.

The transition from newborn to adulthood is a continuum of development, both physically and emotionally. When assessing pediatric patients, keep the child's differences from adults in mind:

The bones of the skull do not close until about 18 months, and joints remain cartilaginous until 5 years.

The child's airway is narrow and will be more quickly and severely obstructed than the adult's. Instead of listening for verbal complaints, note the child's eyes and expression and the degree of activity it takes to distract him from the problem as an indication of its seriousness.

Rib fractures are rare because of the cartilaginous nature of the ribs, though the tissue underneath is more prone to injury.

The liver and spleen are proportionally large and are more subject to injury.

Children are more likely to experience bone injury rather than ligament and tendon injury.

Normal vital signs for children will change through the stages of their development.

Content Self-Evaluation

MULTIPLE CHOICE

_____ 1. A normal pulse quality would be reported as:
  A. 0.   D. 3+.
  B. 1+.   E. 4+.
  C. 2+.

_____ 2. Which of the following is NOT a sign of proximal arterial occlusion?
  A. thrills   D. poor color in the fingertips
  B. pulse deficit   E. slow capillary refill
  C. cold limb

_____ 3. Pitting edema that depresses 1/2 to 1 inch is reported as:
  A. 0.   D. 3+.
  B. 1+.   E. 4+.
  C. 2+.

_____ 4. The pitting of edema will usually disappear within how many seconds after the release of pressure?
  A. 2   D. 8
  B. 4   E. 10
  C. 6

_____ 5. A complete neurologic exam includes which of the following areas?
  A. cranial nerves   D. sensory system
  B. motor system   E. all of the above
  C. reflexes

_____ 6. The cerebral cortex is the center for which of the following?
  A. conscious thought   D. emotions
  B. sensory awareness   E. all of the above
  C. movement

_____ 7. A patient who is drowsy but answers questions is considered to be:
  A. lethargic.   D. comatose.
  B. obtunded.   E. none of the above.
  C. stuporous.

©2009 Pearson Education, Inc.
Paramedic Care: Principles & Practice, Vol. 2, 3rd. Ed.

_____ 8. Normal speech is:
   A. inflected.
   B. clear and strong.
   C. fluent and articulate.
   D. variable in volume.
   E. all of the above.

_____ 9. The term "dysphonia" refers to which of the following?
   A. defective speech caused by motor deficits
   B. voice changes due to vocal cord problems
   C. defective language due to a neurologic problem
   D. voice changes due to aging
   E. none of the above

_____ 10. The term "aphasia" refers to which of the following?
   A. defective speech caused by motor deficits
   B. voice changes due to vocal cord problems
   C. defective language due to a neurologic problem
   D. voice changes due to aging
   E. none of the above

_____ 11. Which of the following is one of the three basic grades of memory?
   A. intermediate
   B. verifiable
   C. redux
   D. remote
   E. retrograde

_____ 12. A question about a patient's wife's birthday tests which of the following types of memory?
   A. intermediate
   B. verifiable
   C. redux
   D. remote
   E. retrograde

_____ 13. During the test of extraoccular eye movement, you should trace which figure in front of your patient's eyes?
   A. an "X"
   B. an "H"
   C. a "1"
   D. a large "O"
   E. any of the above

_____ 14. Stimulation for a blink by touching the eye's surface with fine cotton fibers tests which of the following?
   A. corneal reflex
   B. ptosis
   C. EOM
   D. the trigeminal nerve
   E. none of the above

_____ 15. When a person loses his sense of balance, which cranial nerve has most likely been injured?
   A. equilibrial
   B. glossopharyngeal
   C. acoustic
   D. vagus
   E. accessory

_____ 16. Damage to CN-XII will cause the tongue to deviate in which manner?
   A. downward
   B. upward
   C. toward the side of injury
   D. away from the side of injury
   E. furrowing and curving upward

_____ 17. The pyramidal pathway within the spinal cord mediates which of the following?
   A. voluntary muscle control
   B. involuntary muscle control
   C. dermatome sensation
   D. visceral sensation
   E. vasoconstriction

_____ 18. Damage to the extrapyramidal pathways is likely to cause what type of presentation?
  A. abnormal posture
  B. abnormal gait
  C. involuntary movement
  D. increased muscle tone
  E. all of the above

_____ 19. The twitching of small muscle fibers is:
  A. spasm.
  B. tics.
  C. tremors.
  D. fasciculations.
  E. atrophy.

_____ 20. In cases of muscular dystrophy, the patient's muscles:
  A. increase in size.
  B. decrease in size.
  C. increase in strength.
  D. decrease in strength.
  E. both A and D.

_____ 21. During your testing of a patient's muscle strength, you notice one side to be slightly stronger than the other. This is a normal finding.
  A. True
  B. False

_____ 22. Which of the following procedures describes the Romberg test? Have the patient:
  A. walk heel-to-toe in a straight line.
  B. stand with eyes closed for 20 to 30 seconds.
  C. walk across the room and turn and walk back again.
  D. do a shallow knee bend on each leg in turn.
  E. walk first on his heels, then toes.

_____ 23. An area of skin innervated by a specific peripheral nerve root is a(n):
  A. afferent region.
  B. sensory topographic region.
  C. myotome.
  D. dermatome.
  E. both A and C.

_____ 24. The score on the muscle strength scale that describes a patient able to perform active movement against gravity is:
  A. 5.
  B. 4.
  C. 3.
  D. 2.
  E. 1.

_____ 25. Babinski's response is positive when the sole of the foot is stroked and:
  A. the big toe plantar flexes while other toes dorsiflex.
  B. the big toe plantar flexes while other toes fan out.
  C. the big toe dorsiflexes while other toes fan out.
  D. the big toe dorsiflexes while other toes plantar flex.
  E. all toes plantar flex.

_____ 26. In caring for the ill or injured child, it is important to be which of the following?
  A. confident
  B. direct
  C. honest
  D. calm
  E. all of the above

_____ 27. Children first recognize their parents' faces and voices at about what age?
  A. 2 months
  B. 6 months
  C. 8 months
  D. 10 months
  E. 1 year

_____ 28. Infants begin to sit up at about what age?
  A. 2 to 4 months
  B. 4 to 6 months
  C. 6 to 8 months
  D. 10 months to 1 year
  E. 1 year or later

©2009 Pearson Education, Inc.
Paramedic Care: Principles & Practice, Vol. 2, 3rd. Ed.

_____ 29. The most difficult pediatric age group to assess is the:
A. infant.
B. toddler.
C. preschooler.
D. school-age child.
E. adolescent.

_____ 30. Which of the following groups is particularly distrusting
of strangers?
A. infant
B. toddler
C. preschooler
D. school-age child
E. adolescent

_____ 31. The soft spots in the skull, called fontanelles, close at about what age?
A. 6 months
B. 12 months
C. 18 months
D. 24 months
E. 30 months

_____ 32. Bulging along the sutures of the skull of a young child suggests which
of the following?
A. dehydration
B. reduced venous pressure in the jugular veins
C. decreased arterial pressure
D. arterial blockage to the cerebrum
E. none of the above

_____ 33. Because the tissue of the child's upper airway is so flexible, injuries, infections,
or minor obstructions do not adversely affect it as seriously as they would
an adult's.
A. True
B. False

_____ 34. Which of the following statements regarding the chest of an infant or a small
child is FALSE?
A. Children have a less mobile mediastinum than adults.
B. The chest is rather elastic.
C. The chest is rather flexible.
D. Chest fractures are less likely.
E. The chest comprises more cartilage than the adult's.

_____ 35. Because of the structure of the thoracic cage, the child is less likely to develop tension
pneumothorax than the adult.
A. True
B. False

_____ 36. The normal respiratory rate for an infant is:
A. 30 to 50 breaths per minute.
B. 30 to 60 breaths per minute.
C. 24 to 40 breaths per minute.
D. 22 to 34 breaths per minute.
E. 18 to 30 breaths per minute.

_____ 37. The normal systolic blood pressure for the newborn is:
A. 60 to 90.
B. 87 to 105.
C. 95 to 105.
D. 95 to 110.
E. 112 to 128.

_____ 38. Which of the following is NOT true regarding the abdomen of the child?
A. The liver is proportionally larger than the adult's.
B. The spleen is proportionally larger than the adult's.
C. The abdominal muscles provide less protection than the adult's.
D. The abdomen rarely bulges at the end of inspiration.
E. Inguinal hernias are common in young children.

_____ 39. Which of the following statements is true regarding the recording of examination findings?
   A. The patient care report is only as good as the accuracy, detail, and depth you provide.
   B. The patient chart is a legal document.
   C. The absence of an expected sign in a patient may be just as important as its presence.
   D. The universally accepted organization for recording patient information is SOAP.
   E. All of the above are correct.

_____ 40. The patient's chief complaint is recorded under which element of the SOAP documentation format?
   A. S
   B. O
   C. A
   D. P
   E. none of the above

MATCHING

Match the cranial nerve number with its name and function by writing the appropriate numbers in the spaces provided.

Cranial Nerve	Name	Function
41. I	_____	_____
42. II	_____	_____
43. III	_____	_____
44. IV	_____	_____
45. V	_____	_____
46. VI	_____	_____
47. VII	_____	_____
48. VIII	_____	_____
49. IX	_____	_____
50. X	_____	_____
51. XI	_____	_____
52. XII	_____	_____

Name	Function
A. acoustic	M. smell
B. optic	N. posterior palate and pharynx motor control
C. trochlear	O. trapezius and sternocleidomastoid motor control
D. abducens	P. sight
E. accessory	Q. tongue sensation
F. glossopharyngeal	R. motor control of the tongue
G. trigeminal	S. motor control of the superior oblique muscles
H. oculomotor	T. anterior tongue sensation posterior pharynx motor control
I. vagus	U. lateral rectus muscle motor control
J. hypoglossal	V. hearing and balance
K. facial	W. eye movement and pupil constriction
L. olfactory	X. forehead, cheek, and chin sensation

©2009 Pearson Education, Inc.
Paramedic Care: Principles & Practice, Vol. 2, 3rd. Ed.

Special Project

Physical Assessment—Personal Benchmarking

To perform the physical assessment of a patient, you will need to use the skills of inspection, palpation, auscultation, and percussion. You must not only master each of these skills but also learn to recognize normal and abnormal patient presentations. Often the distinction between normal and abnormal is very small and difficult to recognize without extensive experience. It is also difficult to maintain the ability to differentiate between normal and abnormal signs unless you practice the skill regularly. To help in skills maintenance, use yourself as a physiological model upon which to practice assessment techniques and as a benchmark against which you can measure your patients' responses.

> **Pulse location and evaluation:** Review pages 41 through 42 and 136 through 142.
> *Palpate each of the following arteries for the location, rate, and strength of pulsation.*
> Radial—wrist, thumb side
> Ulnar—wrist, little finger side
> Brachial—medial aspect, just above the elbow
> Carotid—just lateral of the trachea (palpate both)
> Femoral—half the distance between the anterior iliac crest (the bone the belt sits on) and the
>   symphysis pubis (just below the inguinal ligament)
> Popliteal—just behind and below the knee
> Posterior tibial—below the medial malleolus (ankle bone)
> Dorsalis pedis—on top of the foot

Locate each of these pulses on yourself, but realize that you are healthy and perfusing well. It is more difficult to find and evaluate these distal pulses on patients, especially the pulses on the lower extremities and those of patients with serious medical or trauma-induced problems. Remember to place the pads of your fingers lightly over the artery and increase the pressure until you feel the strongest impulse. Rate each pulse from 0 to 3+ (with 0 = absent, 1+ = weak or thready, 2+ = normal, 3+ = bounding). Practice finding and rating the pulses quickly. These skills will be invaluable when you go to assess your patients.

You might try counting a pulse in your arm or forearm while driving or riding in a car. The vibration of travel makes the task much harder and simulates pulse evaluation in a moving ambulance. It might also be helpful to assess the pulses of friends and fellow emergency care workers to gain invaluable practice.

Auscultation Exercise

Indicate the proper locations at which to auscultate heart sounds on the accompanying illustration. Be sure to include locations for auscultation of sounds in the aortic, pulmonic, mitral, and tricuspid areas as well as the point of maximal impulse.

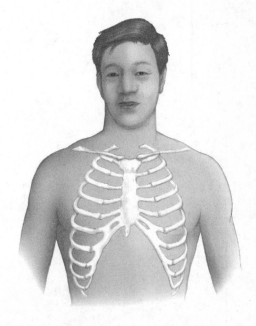

3

Patient Assessment in the Field

Because Chapter 3 is lengthy, it has been divided into sections to aid your study. Read the assigned text pages; then progress through the objectives and self-evaluation materials as you would with other chapters. When you feel confident of your grasp of the content, proceed to the next section.

Section I, pp. 183–211

Review of Chapter Objectives

After reading this chapter, you should be able to:

1. Recognize hazards/potential hazards associated with the medical and trauma scene. **pp. 187–194**

During the scene size-up, you must examine the scene before you arrive at the patient's side. It is a time to evaluate and prepare for hazards, including blood, fluids, airborne pathogens, and other conditions that may threaten your life or health. These conditions include the hazards of fire, structural collapse, traffic, unstable surfaces, electricity, broken glass, or jagged metal. Hazardous materials can involve chemical spills, radiation, and toxic environments. Finally, scene hazards can also include violent, disturbed, or unruly bystanders or patients. These hazards are not limited to the trauma scene but may be found at many medical scenes as well.

2. Identify unsafe scenes and describe methods for making them safe. **pp. 187–194**

Your responsibility at the emergency scene is to recognize hazards, including fire, structural collapse, traffic, unstable surfaces, electricity, broken glass, jagged metal, and hazardous materials and then act appropriately to protect yourself, other rescuers, and your patient. Unless you are specially trained and equipped to handle a specific hazard, do not enter the scene. In most cases, you will rely on the fire department, rescue service, police department, power company, hazmat team, or other specially trained personnel to secure the scene before you enter. If there is ever a question of whether a scene is safe or unsafe, do not enter the scene.

3. Discuss common mechanisms of injury/nature of illness. **pp. 196–198**

Trauma is induced by a mechanism of injury through which forces enter the body and do physical harm. Common mechanisms include blunt trauma—for example, vehicle crashes (auto, recreational, watercraft, and bicycle), pedestrian vs. vehicle impacts, and falls—and penetrating trauma—for example, gunshot and knife wounds. Medical problems have a related cause called the nature of the illness. The scene can provide evidence as to the nature of the illness. Examples include the presence of nebulizers, which suggest asthma; drug paraphernalia, which suggest overdose; and medications, which suggest preexisting cardiac or other problems.

4. Predict patterns of injury based on mechanism of injury. pp. 196–197, 211–213

Analyze the strength, direction, and nature of the forces expressed to the patient during the incident. This analysis will suggest the probable type of injury, the organs involved, and the seriousness of the injury. In a vehicle crash, for example, such things as a broken windshield, a bent steering wheel, an intrusion into the passenger compartment, and the use of restraints by occupants can suggest potential injuries and their severity. Types of injuries can also be predicted for each type of vehicle crash—frontal, lateral, rear-end, rotational, and rollover. The analysis of the accident can lead to your anticipation of possible injuries or to an index of suspicion.

5. Discuss the reason for identifying the total number of patients at the scene. pp. 195–196

Determining the number of patients at a scene is important to ensure that the needed resources are summoned to the scene and that every patient is cared for. At every scene, you should ask yourself, "Could there be others who are injured or ill?" At the trauma scene, it is common to find a patient wandering among the bystanders; however, the medical scene can have "hidden patients," too. The wife of a cardiac arrest patient, for example, may herself become a patient because of the emotional stress of the incident. Knowing the number of patients can help you gauge whether on-scene resources are adequate or whether you need to request that additional units and manpower be dispatched to the scene. The earlier this request is made, the quicker those resources will arrive.

6. Organize the management of a scene following size-up. pp. 195–196

The management of the scene following the scene size-up includes requesting both the appropriate units and the personnel to manage scene hazards and the appropriate number and care levels of ambulances and personnel to treat the patients. You must also take the necessary steps to ensure overall scene safety and to protect yourself, the patient, other scene personnel, and bystanders. The scene size-up also prepares you to manage the care of the patient by helping you recognize the mechanism of injury and anticipate injuries (index of suspicion) or by recognizing the nature of the illness.

7. Explain the reasons for identifying the need for additional help or assistance during the scene size-up. pp. 190–196

Multiple patients at the emergency scene can rapidly overwhelm your ability to provide effective care. If you wait until you are at a patient's side before calling for additional help, you may be distracted from making the call and delay an effective response. In cases in which the number of patients far outstrips your ability to provide care, you may need to initiate a mass casualty response.

8. Summarize the reasons for forming a general impression of the patient. pp. 196–199

The initial general impression of your patient takes into account the patient's age, gender, race, and other factors that will help you determine the seriousness of the problem and establish your priorities for patient care and transport. As you learn more about the patient through the primary survey and the focused history and physical assessment, you will refine and improve on the accuracy and depth of the general impression. As you develop your general impression of the patient early in the assessment process, you also can begin to establish a rapport with him, explaining why you are there, describing what will be happening to him, and giving the patient the opportunity to refuse care.

9. Discuss methods of assessing mental status/levels of consciousness in the adult, child, and infant patient. pp. 200–201

Initially determine the patient's mental status by categorizing him according to the AVPU system. Using this method, the patient is classified either Alert, responsive to Verbal stimuli, responsive to

©2009 Pearson Education, Inc.
Paramedic Care: Principles & Practice, Vol. 2, 3rd. Ed.

Painful stimuli, or Unresponsive. You can further refine the evaluation by questioning the patient to determine orientation to place, time, and person and by differentiating his response to pain into purposeful and purposeless movement and decerebrate and decorticate posturing. An alert response for the infant or child is difficult to assess because of that patient's limited speech capabilities. Evaluate pediatric patients for activity and curiosity, being aware that a quiet child is often a seriously ill or injured one.

10. Discuss methods of assessing and securing the airway in the adult, child, and infant patient. pp. 201–206

The patient who is speaking clearly (or the child or infant who is crying loudly) has a patent airway. For other patients, position your head at the patient's mouth and look, listen, and feel for air moving through the airway. If you detect no movement, open the airway by using either the jaw-thrust (in patients with trauma and suspected spine injury) or the head-tilt/chin-lift maneuver. Suction any fluids from the airway and remove obstructions using the Heimlich maneuver or laryngoscopy with Magill forceps. Secure the airway, as needed, with an oral or a nasal airway, endotracheal intubation, or creation of a needle or surgical airway. When you have a pediatric patient, be sure to position the head and neck properly (using slight extension and padding under the shoulders), taking into account the differences in the pediatric anatomy. Also, reduce the size of the airways, laryngoscope blades, and endotracheal tubes you use with these patients.

11. State reasons for cervical spine management for the trauma patient. p. 199

The spinal cord is the major communication, distribution, and collection conduit for the central nervous system. It is protected by the spinal column, the bony and flexible structure that runs from the base of the skull to just below the pelvis. If the column is injured, it may become unstable and permit injury to the spinal cord. Because injuries to the cord have such serious consequences, you should immobilize the spine early in your assessment and take care to protect this essential communication pathway. Its immobilization will not harm the patient, whereas uncontrolled movement can cause permanent spinal cord injury.

12. Analyze a scene to determine if spinal precautions are required. pp. 196–197, 211–213

Your examination of the scene and the analysis of the mechanism of injury will suggest or rule out the potential for spinal injury. The patient with a significant mechanism of injury—a severe vehicle crash; a fall from a high point injury, causing a major long bone fracture; or any injury or mechanism of injury that suggests the body was subjected to significant trauma forces—has a likelihood of spinal fracture and requires spinal precautions.

13. Describe methods for assessing respiration in the adult, child, and infant patient. pp. 206–207

If your patient is speaking clearly (or if an infant or a child patient is crying loudly) presume the airway is clear. Otherwise, listen for the sounds of airway restriction or obstruction, such as gurgling, stridor, or wheezes. If airway sounds are absent, place your ear at the patient's mouth while you listen, watch, and feel for air movement through it. If there is any doubt about airway patency, position the head with the jaw-thrust or head-tilt/chin-lift maneuver. With a child, do not hyperextend the neck, because this may block the airway. You may have to place padding behind the shoulders of a small child or an infant to maintain proper head positioning.

14. Describe the methods used to locate and assess a pulse in the adult, child, and infant patient. pp. 207–210

Use the pads of your fingers and apply gentle, increasing pressure until you feel a strong pulsing over the radial artery in the adult and brachial artery in the small child or infant. If the radial or brachial pulse cannot be felt, check the carotid or, in the infant, the apical pulse. An adult radial pulse generally suggests a blood pressure of at least 80 mmHg; a carotid pulse suggests a systolic blood pressure of at least 60 mmHg. Pulse rates usually decrease with age from a high of 100 to 180 in the infant to 60 to 100 in the adult. The pulse should be strong and regular.

15. **Discuss the need for assessing the patient for external bleeding.**   p. 207

The patient with the potential for external hemorrhage must be assessed to determine both the nature and the extent of the blood loss. Any significant external hemorrhage must be halted and the amount of loss approximated to help prevent hypovolemia and to determine what effects the loss will have on the patient's body.

16. **Describe normal and abnormal findings when assessing skin color, temperature, and condition.**   p. 207

Normal skin is warm, moist, and pink in color (in light-skinned people), reflecting good perfusion. The body's compensation for shock results in vasoconstriction, which produces mottled, cyanotic, pale, or ashen skin color and skin that is cool to the touch. Capillary refill times may exceed 3 seconds, though this may be due to a number of preexisting conditions in adults.

17. **Explain the reason and process for prioritizing a patient for care and transport.**   pp. 210–211

At the conclusion of the primary survey, you must determine your patient's priority, which will indicate how to proceed with assessment, care, and transport. With a seriously ill or injured patient, perform a rapid head-to-toe assessment. With a stable medical or trauma patient, perform a focused history and physical exam. You will also need to determine the priority for transport—either immediate transport with care rendered en route or with most care provided at the scene followed by transport.

18. **Use the findings of the initial survey to determine the patient's perfusion status.**   pp. 207–210

The primary survey provides you with a general impression of the patient, a determination of the patient's mental status, and an evaluation of the airway, breathing, and circulation. This information indicates the status of the patient's respiration/oxygenation and circulation. It also indicates the patient's level of consciousness and the perfusion of the body's most important end-organ, the brain.

Case Study Review

Reread the case study on pages 183 and 184 in Paramedic Care: Patient Assessment *and then read the following discussion.*

This case study gives you the opportunity quickly to identify and review the elements of the patient assessment process. The process involves the scene size-up, primary survey, focused history and physical exam, detailed exam, and ongoing assessments.

Even before Chris arrives at the scene, she uses the time available to her to review the elements of the scene size-up and her expected assessment and care. She identifies the likely mechanism of injury as a fall from a great height with an impact on an unforgiving surface. She suspects very serious injuries and the need for rapid assessment and care. Given the expected mechanism of injury, Chris may alert the trauma center to let them know of the incident and, if she is more than 20 minutes away from the center, might also put the helicopter service on standby.

As Chris arrives, she sizes up the scene and quickly determines that the dispatch information was correct. She dons her gloves to protect against the dangers of body substance contamination and requests additional help from the fire department. She also recognizes that this is not likely to be a hazardous scene but that she may have to contend with curious onlookers and those who are made emotionally distraught by the sight of blood and gore. Finally, Chris considers the mechanism of injury to help her anticipate injuries. Given the circumstances, Chris expects numerous broken bones, internal injuries, and head and spine trauma in this patient.

As Chris moves to the patient's side, she begins the initial assessment. She already has a general impression of the patient's condition, and it is not good. She builds upon this impression as the assessment continues. She immediately directs an EMT to hold cervical spine stabilization as one of the first steps

©2009 Pearson Education, Inc.
Paramedic Care: Principles & Practice, Vol. 2, 3rd. Ed.

in the initial assessment. He continues manual stabilization until the patient is fully immobilized by mechanical means later on. Chris determines the patient is completely unresponsive and then moves to assess the ABCs. The airway is cleared, respirations are supported, and Chris begins treating the patient for shock. These actions are essential to sustain life, and Chris does not delay her primary assessment to care for any nonlife-threatening injuries.

With the airway, breathing, and circulation stabilized, Chris moves to the rapid trauma assessment. Here she concentrates her patient evaluation on possible critical injuries. She examines the head, neck, chest, abdomen, pelvis, and extremities and notes the depressed skull fracture, deformed thorax, rigid abdomen, and pelvic and femur fractures. She also notes pertinent negatives (expected but not substantiated findings), such as the absent signs of pneumothorax. Since this is a critical trauma patient, transport and life-sustaining interventions are the highest priorities, and Chris does not perform a detailed physical exam. Doing so would extend the time at the scene and probably not suggest any care steps that Chris and Nick are not already planning. The care team determine that their patient is in critical condition and needs the services of a trauma center. They make arrangements to expedite transport.

Once the patient is on the way to the trauma center and all critical interventions have been performed, Chris provides a reassessment. She quickly reevaluates the level of responsiveness, ABCs, vital signs, and signs and symptoms. She documents the results to track the patient's progress during her care—is the patient improving, deteriorating, or remaining the same? Since the patient is critical, Chris performs the ongoing assessment every 5 minutes. (She would perform it every 15 minutes or so for a nonserious patient.) She also employs the reassessment whenever her team performs an invasive procedure or anytime they notice a change in a patient sign or symptom.

Content Self-Evaluation

MULTIPLE CHOICE

_____ 1. As a paramedic, you will certainly never perform a comprehensive history and physical exam in the acute setting.
A. True
B. False

_____ 2. Which component of the patient assessment process will be performed during patient transport?
A. scene survey
B. primary survey
C. focused history and physical exam
D. detailed physical exam
E. ongoing assessment

_____ 3. After the scene size-up and if necessary, you should inform the dispatcher of:
A. the nature of the medical or trauma emergency.
B. what resources you need.
C. the phone number at which you can be reached.
D. what actions you and your crew are taking.
E. all of the above except C.

_____ 4. Which of the following is NOT a component of the scene size-up?
A. standard precautions
B. general impression of the patient
C. location of all patients
D. mechanism of injury/nature of the illness analysis
E. scene safety

_____ 5. Which of the following standard precautions devices will you employ with every patient you treat?
A. latex or vinyl gloves
B. protective eyewear
C. face mask
D. gown
E. both B and C

_____ 6. Whenever you plan to intubate a patient, you should wear:
   A. latex or vinyl gloves and a gown.
   B. protective eyewear, a gown, and a face mask.
   C. latex or vinyl gloves, protective eyewear, and a face mask.
   D. protective eyewear and a gown.
   E. latex or vinyl gloves.

_____ 7. The HEPA respirator is designed to filter out which of the following pathogens that may be encountered when providing prehospital emergency care?
   A. tuberculosis
   B. smallpox
   C. anthrax
   D. flu
   E. tetanus toxoid

_____ 8. The intent of the safety analysis portion of the scene survey is to ensure the safety of:
   A. the patient.
   B. bystanders.
   C. fellow responders.
   D. yourself.
   E. all of the above.

_____ 9. To handle a scene safety issue properly, you must be:
   A. properly trained.
   B. properly equipped.
   C. properly clothed.
   D. prepared to attempt rescue procedures in which you have not been trained.
   E. A, B, and C.

_____ 10. Potential hazards to rule out before entering the scene include all of the following EXCEPT:
   A. fire.
   B. electrocution.
   C. contamination with blood.
   D. structural collapse.
   E. broken glass and jagged metal.

_____ 11. When called to a shooting or domestic disturbance, until the police arrive and secure the scene you should remain:
   A. a few blocks away.
   B. outside the residence.
   C. just down the street.
   D. at the door but do not enter.
   E. either B or C.

_____ 12. At which of the following incidents would you NOT expect to discover more than one patient in your scene size-up?
   A. a two-car collision
   B. a carbon monoxide poisoning in a home
   C. a car crash in which a child seat and diaper bag are visible
   D. a fall out of a tree
   E. a hazardous materials spill in a high school chemistry lab

_____ 13. You should delay the call for additional ambulances until you begin your initial survey because you will not have enough information to determine the needs of the scene until then.
   A. True
   B. False

_____ 14. The two important functions that must begin immediately in the mass casualty situation are:
   A. triage and incident management.
   B. rescue and triage.
   C. firefighting and rescue.
   D. incident management and extrication.
   E. incident management and scene isolation.

©2009 Pearson Education, Inc.
Paramedic Care: Principles & Practice, Vol. 2, 3rd. Ed.

15. The responsibilities of incident management at a disaster scene include all of the following EXCEPT:
    A. performing a scene size-up.
    B. triaging initial patients for care.
    C. determining the need for additional resources.
    D. radioing for additional equipment and personnel.
    E. directing incoming crews.

16. The responsibilities of the triage person at the disaster scene include all of the following EXCEPT:
    A. determining a patient's priority for immediate transport.
    B. determining a patient's priority for delayed transport.
    C. performing simple but lifesaving procedures.
    D. providing intensive care on salvageable patients.
    E. all of the above.

17. The mechanism of injury analysis examines:
    A. body locations affected.
    B. strength of the crash forces.
    C. direction of the crash forces.
    D. nature of the crash forces.
    E. all of the above.

18. The index of suspicion is best defined as:
    A. patient priority for care based on the MOI.
    B. anticipation of the nature of forces involved in an accident.
    C. prediction of injuries based on the MOI.
    D. prediction of degree of injury based on the patient's appearance.
    E. none of the above.

19. The nature of the illness is determined from information you receive from:
    A. the patient.
    B. the patient's family.
    C. bystanders.
    D. scene clues.
    E. all of the above.

20. The initial survey includes all of the following EXCEPT:
    A. forming a general impression of the patient.
    B. stabilizing the cervical spine as needed.
    C. immobilizing fractures.
    D. assessing the airway.
    E. assessing the circulation.

21. The general patient impression is based on all of the following EXCEPT:
    A. blood pressure.
    B. mechanism of injury.
    C. chief complaint.
    D. the environment.
    E. your instincts.

22. Which of the following is NOT a purpose served by your initial introduction to the patient?
    A. identifying yourself
    B. identifying your reason for being there
    C. establishing your level of training
    D. giving the patient an opportunity to refuse care
    E. establishing informed consent

23. During the initial survey, the cervical spine should be stabilized:
    A. after the airway is established.
    B. just before you attempt artificial ventilation.
    C. immediately, if suggested by the MOI.
    D. after the circulation check.
    E. as the last step of the primary survey.

_____ 24. Which of the following conditions does NOT normally cause an altered mental status?
- A. eupnea
- B. drug overdose
- C. head injury
- D. poisoning
- E. sepsis

_____ 25. A patient who moves only his arm when firmly pinched between the thumb and first finger and shows no other responses will be classified as which of the following under the AVPU system?
- A. A
- B. V
- C. P
- D. U
- E. cannot be determined with the information at hand

_____ 26. A patient who is disoriented and confused would be classified as which of the following under the AVPU system?
- A. A
- B. V
- C. P
- D. U
- E. cannot be determined with the information at hand

_____ 27. Stridor can usually be caused by all of the following EXCEPT:
- A. infection.
- B. gastric distress.
- C. foreign body.
- D. severe swelling.
- E. allergic reaction.

_____ 28. For stridor that is caused by respiratory burns, the care procedure most likely to maintain the airway is:
- A. suctioning.
- B. blow-by oxygen and a quiet ride to the hospital.
- C. a surgical airway.
- D. early endotracheal intubation.
- E. vasoconstrictor medications.

_____ 29. A patient with abnormally deep respirations is said to be:
- A. hyperpneic.
- B. tachypneic.
- C. eupneic.
- D. bradypneic.
- E. hypopneic.

_____ 30. The presence of a radial pulse suggests that the systolic blood pressure is at least:
- A. 60 mmHg.
- B. 70 mmHg.
- C. 80 mmHg.
- D. 100 mmHg.
- E. 120 mmHg.

LISTING

List the components of patient assessment in the field.

31. _____

32. _____

33. _____

34. _____

35. _____

©2009 Pearson Education, Inc.
Paramedic Care: Principles & Practice, Vol. 2, 3rd. Ed.

Special Project

Scene Size-Up Exercise

Review the accompanying photographs and identify the likely hazards you should suspect at each scene.

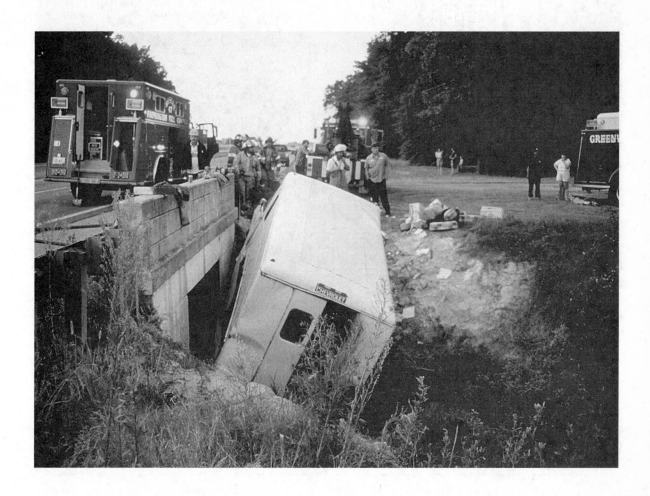

A. _____

_____

_____

_____

_____

_____

_____

_____

_____

_____

_____

_____

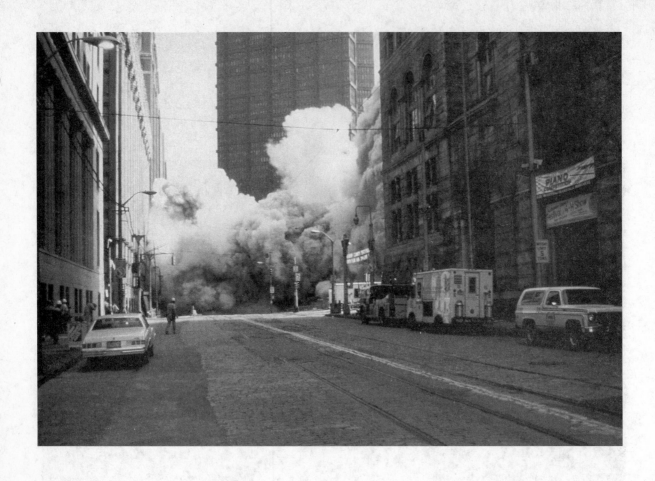

B. _____
_____
_____
_____
_____
_____
_____
_____
_____
_____
_____
_____

©2009 Pearson Education, Inc.
Paramedic Care: Principles & Practice, Vol. 2, 3rd. Ed.

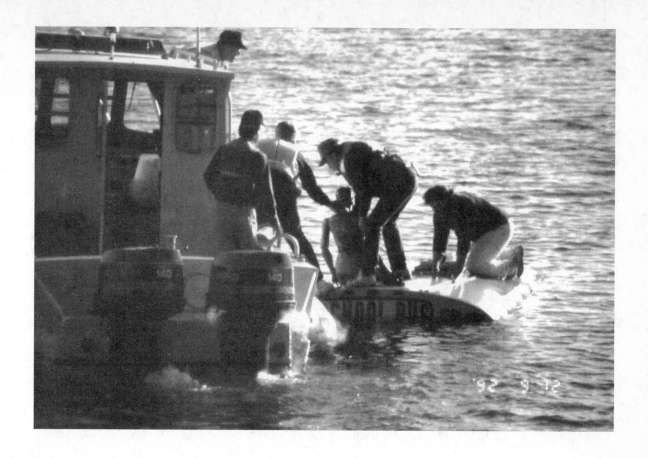

C. _____
_____
_____
_____
_____
_____
_____
_____
_____
_____
_____
_____
_____

Review of Chapter Objectives

After reading this chapter, you should be able to:

19. Describe orthostatic vital signs and evaluate their usefulness in assessing a patient in shock.   **p. 228**

The test for orthostatic vital signs, also called the tilt test, evaluates vital signs (blood pressure and pulse rate) before and after moving the patient from the supine to the seated, then to the full standing position. If after 30 to 60 seconds either the blood pressure drops by more than 10 mmHg or the pulse rate rises by more than 10, consider the test positive and suspect hypovolemia. (Note that the change in pulse rate is the more sensitive indicator.) Do not use this test when other indicators of shock are present because it places stress on the cardiovascular system.

20. Describe the medical patient physical examination.   **pp. 223–231**

The medical patient physical exam evaluates the head, ears, eyes, nose, and throat (HEENT); chest; abdomen; pelvis; extremities; posterior surface; and vital signs, discretely looking for illness or disease signs. The exam may be modified to meet the specific patient complaints of chest pain, respiratory distress, altered mental status, and acute abdomen. The medical patient exam may also include the results of pulse oximetry, as well as cardiac and glucose level monitoring.

21. Differentiate among the assessment for unresponsive, altered mental status, and alert medical patients.   **pp. 222–231**

Responsive and unresponsive medical patients are examined in much different fashions. The *responsive patient* can provide information regarding his chief complaint, history of the present illness, past medical history, and current health status. This information, along with a physical exam focused on the areas of expected signs, provides the information necessary to make a field diagnosis.

The *unresponsive patient* cannot provide this information, and the caregiver must garner it from family and bystanders and through a more intensive and comprehensive physical examination.

The *patient with an altered mental status* is assessed like the unresponsive patient, though some information may be obtained from the patient. The information may not be reliable, hence the need for a more comprehensive physical exam.

22. Discuss the reasons for reconsidering the mechanism of injury.   **pp. 211–213**

After the primary survey and rapid trauma assessments or focused history and physical exam, you have gathered enough information about your patient to determine if the mechanism of injury (and your resulting index of suspicion for associated injuries) agrees with your assessment findings. If it does, maintain your priority for care and transport. If they do not agree, reevaluate your index of suspicion and the physical findings and possibly adjust your patient's priority. If you do alter your patient's priority, always err on the side of precaution.

23. Recite examples and explain why patients should receive a rapid trauma assessment.   **p. 213**

Every patient with a significant mechanism of injury, an altered level of consciousness, or multiple body-system traumas should receive the rapid trauma assessment. These patients are likely to have serious internal injuries and/or hemorrhage. However, the signs and symptoms of serious injury and shock are often hidden by other, more gruesome or painful injuries or by the body's compensatory

©2009 Pearson Education, Inc.
Paramedic Care: Principles & Practice, Vol. 2, 3rd. Ed.

mechanisms. Without maintaining a high index of suspicion for serious injury and evaluating the patient via the rapid trauma assessment, you are likely to overlook the patient with serious and life-threatening injury.

24. Describe the trauma patient physical examination. pp. 213–221

The physical assessment of the trauma patient begins during the primary survey with the check of the ABCs and then branches to either the rapid trauma assessment or the focused history and physical exam. The patient with a serious mechanism of injury, altered mental status, or multi-system trauma receives a rapid trauma assessment, a fast, systematic physical exam evaluating body regions where serious or life-threatening problems are likely to occur. This assessment is a rapid evaluation of the critical structures and regions of the head (HEENT), neck, chest, abdomen, pelvis, extremities, posterior body, and vital signs. The patient with isolated trauma has an assessment directed at the areas of expected injury or patient complaint.

25. Describe the elements of the rapid trauma assessment and discuss their evaluation. pp. 213–221

Each region of the body is inspected, palpated, and, as appropriate, auscultated and percussed to identify the signs of injury (DCAP-BTLS and crepitus). For each region, the specific assessment considerations include the actions listed in the following discussion.

Evaluate the *head* for any signs of serious bleeding and deformity from skull fracture. Also check for discharge from the ears and nose, for the stability of the facial bones, and for the patency of the airway.

Evaluate the *neck* for lacerations involving the major blood vessels and serious hemorrhage and possible air embolism. Examine the jugular veins for abnormal distention and palpate the position and any unusual motion of the trachea. Also examine for subcutaneous emphysema and then any evidence of spinal trauma.

Evaluate the *chest* for signs of respiratory distress, including the use of accessory muscles and retractions, and any signs of open wounds. Also observe the motion of the chest. Chest excursion should be bilaterally equal and symmetrical. Palpate for signs of clavicular or costal fracture and subcutaneous emphysema. Erythema may be present, but the frank ecchymotic discoloration of a contusion takes time to develop. Auscultate the lungs at the midaxillary line for bilaterally equal breath sounds.

Evaluate the *abdomen* for exaggerated abdominal wall motion, and inspect and palpate for signs of injury, noting rigidity, guarding, tenderness, and rebound tenderness.

Evaluate the *pelvis* for signs of injury and apply pressure directed posteriorly and medially to the iliac crests and pressure directed posteriorly to the symphysis pubis to check for pelvic instability.

Evaluate the *extremities* for signs of injury, distal circulation, and innervation.

Evaluate the *posterior body* for signs of injury, and be especially watchful for potential signs of spinal injury.

Evaluate *vital signs*, first to establish a baseline and then to obtain other readings to compare to that baseline. Evaluate direct pupil response to light during the rapid trauma assessment, but evaluate the other pupillary responses during more specific and directed evaluation.

Gather a patient *history* while you perform the rapid trauma assessment. This should include the elements of the SAMPLE assessment (Signs/Symptoms, Allergies, Medications, Past medical history, Last oral intake, and Events preceding the incident).

26. Identify cases when the rapid assessment is suspended to provide patient care. pp. 213–218

The rapid trauma assessment is interrupted to provide patient care whenever you identify any life-threatening condition that can be quickly addressed. Just as you would suction the airway when you find it full of fluids during the primary survey, you might provide pleural decompression during the rapid trauma assessment when you notice a developing tension pneumothorax. You might also administer oxygen to a patient who begins to display dyspnea and accessory muscle use during your chest examination. Other examples include employing the PASG for the patient with the early signs of shock compensation and an unstable pelvic fracture found during the pelvic assessment or immediate provision of spinal immobilization upon noticing a neurologic deficit during the extremity exam.

27. Discuss the reason for performing a focused history and physical exam. pp. 211, 224, 230

The focused history and physical exam is the third step (following the scene size-up and primary survery) of the patient assessment process. It is an assessment directed at the areas where the signs of serious injury or illness are expected. It also draws upon a quick history to identify information supporting a specific diagnosis and elements critical to the continued care of the patient. The focused history and physical exam takes you quickly toward determining the nature of the illness or the existence of serious and specific injuries. It is performed in different ways for trauma patients with significant injuries or mechanisms of injury, trauma patients with isolated injuries, responsive medical patients, and unresponsive medical patients.

28. Describe when and why a detailed physical examination is necessary. pp. 231–232

The detailed assessment is a combination of a detailed history and a comprehensive physical exam either to identify or to learn more about the effects of an illness or injury on the body. It, in its entirety, is employed only when all other assessment and care procedures have been performed, most likely during transport to the hospital and then only for patients with serious trauma or disease. Since seriously ill or injured patients require constant care, this assessment is rarely performed in the prehospital setting. However, portions of the detailed physical exam are frequently employed to examine specific body regions, looking for expected signs of illness or injury.

29. Discuss the components of the detailed physical examination. pp. 232–238

The detailed physical exam involves a comprehensive evaluation of each body region using the skills of inspection, palpation, auscultation, and percussion. It begins at the head, progresses downward to the extremities, and includes the regions discussed in the following section.

Head. Inspect and palpate for any skull or facial asymmetry, deformity, instability, tenderness, unusual warmth, or crepitus. Look for the development of Battle's sign and periorbital ecchymosis.

Eyes. Carefully inspect the eye for shape, size, coloration, and foreign bodies, as well as pupillary equality, light reactivity, consensual movement, and visual acuity.

Ears. Examine the external ear for signs of injury and the ear canal for hemorrhage or discharge.

Nose and sinuses. Palpate the external aspect of the nose and examine the nares for signs of injury, hemorrhage, discharge, and flaring. The nasal mucosa is rich in vasculature and may bleed heavily.

Mouth and pharynx. Examine the oral cavity for signs of injury and the potential for airway compromise. Notice any fluids or odors and examine tongue movement for signs of cranial nerve injury.

Neck. Briefly inspect the neck for signs of injury, with special attention to open wounds and possible severe hemorrhage and air embolism. Palpate the trachea to identify any unusual movement and examine for jugular vein distention.

Chest and lungs. Observe the patient's breathing for symmetrical chest movement and respiratory pattern. Note any accessory muscle use, and auscultate and percuss for unusual findings. Look for signs of injury, and palpate for crepitus and tenderness.

Cardiovascular system. Look to the skin for pallor, and palpate a pulse for rate, rhythm, and strength. Auscultate for heart sounds, and locate the point of maximal impulse.

Abdomen. Inspect and palpate for signs of injury and rebound tenderness, rigidity, and guarding.

Pelvis. Observe the area; then place medial and posterior pressure on the iliac crests and posterior pressure on the symphysis pubis.

©2009 Pearson Education, Inc.
Paramedic Care: Principles & Practice, Vol. 2, 3rd. Ed.

Genitalia. As needed, examine these organs for hemorrhage and, in the male, priapism.

Anus and rectum. If hemorrhage is present, inspect the anus and rectum and apply direct pressure to halt bleeding.

Peripheral vascular system. Inspect all four extremities, observing and palpating for signs of injury and skin color, moisture, temperature, and capillary refill to ensure distal circulation.

Musculoskeletal system. Palpate the musculature of the extremities, feeling for differences in muscle tone and the flexibility and the active and passive range of motion in joints.

Nervous system. Evaluate the nervous system by examining the following:

- **Mental status and speech.** Assess the patient's level of consciousness and orientation and compare these findings to earlier ones. Note the patient's speech patterns, appropriateness of dress, and actions.
- **Cranial nerves.** Test the discrete cranial nerves that have not already been tested.
- **Motor system.** Inspect the patient's general body structure, positioning, muscular development, and coordination.
- **Sensory system.** Test for ability to sense pain, touch, position, temperature, and vibration over the extremities and, as necessary, the dermatomes.
- **Reflexes.** Test deep tendon reflexes with a reflex hammer, noting heightened or diminished responses. Test superficial abdominal reflexes and plantar response.

Vital signs. Repeat the evaluation of the vital signs, including blood pressure, pulse, respiration, temperature, and pupillary response.

30. Explain what additional care is provided while performing the detailed physical exam. pp. 232–238

Since the complete detailed physical exam is an elective assessment, anytime a significant sign of injury or the patient's condition suggests a care step, perform that step. The same principle applies when a portion of the comprehensive physical exam is performed on a discrete body region as a part of the focused history and physical exam.

31. Distinguish between the detailed physical exam that is performed on a trauma patient and that on the medical patient. pp. 232–238

The detailed physical exam for the trauma patient focuses evaluation on the areas where signs of injury are expected based on the mechanism of injury analysis or the patient's complaints (for example, examination for signs of anterior chest injury when an auto steering wheel is deformed). The detailed physical exam for the medical patient is directed to the areas of patient complaint, as well as those areas where the signs of an expected illness might be found (for example, an examination for pitting edema in the dependent areas with the congestive heart failure patient). The history component of the assessment also differs with trauma and medical patients. With the trauma patient, you may gather an abbreviated (SAMPLE) history, while, with the medical patient, you may perform a more in-depth history evaluation as described in Chapter 1, "The History."

32. Differentiate between patients requiring a detailed physical exam and those who do not. pp. 231–232

The patients who receive a complete detailed physical exam are patients with serious medical or trauma injuries. They receive the detailed physical exam during transport to the hospital after other important care measures have been employed. They represent a very small percentage of patients whom you will treat because seriously ill or injured patients often require almost continuous care. *Portions* of the detailed exam will, however, be performed on many patients, and these portions will be directed at a body region where signs of injury or illness are expected. Patients receiving portions of the detailed exam include those with isolated injuries and those with stable medical problems. Seriously ill or injured patients may receive a detailed exam aimed at discovering significant signs of the pathology generally associated with cardiac, respiratory, vascular, abdominal, musculoskeletal, or nervous system problems.

33. Discuss the rationale for repeating the primary survey as part of the ongoing assessment. pp. 238–240

The primary survey, with its examination of mental status and evaluation of the airway, breathing, and circulation, contains crucial elements of continuing patient assessment. These components of the primary survey can quickly tell you when the patient is suffering from a life-threatening or serious problem and can help you monitor the patient's need for care. For this reason, these components are an integral part of any ongoing assessment.

34. Describe the components of the ongoing assessment. pp. 236–241

The components of the ongoing assessment include reassessment of the pertinent elements of the primary survey, focused history and physical exam or rapid trauma assessment, and vital signs and include the following:

Mental status. Quickly reevaluate the patient's mental status to determine AVPU status or level of orientation.

Airway patency/breathing rate and quality. Perform a quick check of airway patency and breathing rate, volume, and quality to ensure respiration is adequate.

Pulse rate and quality. Quickly reevaluate the pulse rate, strength, and regularity to ensure they remain within normal limits.

Skin condition. Quickly check the skin for moisture, temperature, and capillary refill to monitor distal perfusion.

Vital signs. Reassess blood pressure and temperature (along with pulse and respiration) and compare to baseline findings to determine whether the patient's condition is improving, deteriorating, or remaining the same.

Focused assessment. Quickly reevaluate the signs of injury/illness to identify any changes. This may include reevaluating pertinent negatives to rule out an evolving problem.

Effects of interventions. Repeat the ongoing assessment soon after any major intervention to determine the intervention's impact on the patient's condition.

Transport priorities. Based on the findings of the ongoing assessment, either confirm or modify the patient's priority for care and transport.

35. Describe trending of assessment components. pp. 238–241

Trending of the elements of the ongoing assessment—comparing of sequential findings—will suggest whether your patient's condition is improving, deteriorating, or remaining the same. This information prompts you to modify your priorities for patient care and transport and may ultimately cause you to modify your field diagnosis.

36. Discuss medical identification devices/systems. p. 220

Examine the patient's wrists, ankles, and neck for medical alert jewelry reflecting preexisting medical conditions, such as diabetes, epilepsy, allergies, and use of medications. Also check the wallet or purse for such information. This information may help you and the emergency department in prescribing care for the patient.

37. Given several preprogrammed and moulaged medical and trauma patients, provide the appropriate scene survey, initial assessment, focused assessment, detailed assessment, and ongoing assessments. pp. 186–241

During your classroom, clinical, and field training, you will assess real and simulated patients and develop management plans for them. Use the information presented in this text chapter, the information on patient assessment in the field presented by your instructors, and the guidance given by your clinical and field preceptors to develop good patient assessment skills. Continue to refine these skills once your training ends and you begin your career as a paramedic.

©2009 Pearson Education, Inc.
Paramedic Care: Principles & Practice, Vol. 2, 3rd. Ed.

Content Self-Evaluation

MULTIPLE CHOICE

_____ 1. The focused history and physical exam are conducted differently for the four different categories of patients. Which of the following is NOT one of those categories?
   A. responsive medical patient
   B. unresponsive medical patient
   C. pediatric patient with altered consciousness
   D. trauma patient with an isolated injury
   E. trauma patient with a significant mechanism of injury

_____ 2. Which of the following is NOT a mechanism of injury that calls for rapid transport to the trauma center?
   A. ejection from a vehicle
   B. vehicle rollover
   C. severe vehicle deformity in a high-speed crash
   D. fall from less than 20 feet
   E. bicycle collision with loss of consciousness

_____ 3. The decision to provide rapid transport of a patient to the trauma center is predicated upon either the mechanism of injury or the:
   A. blood pressure reading.   D. ongoing assessments.
   B. physical signs of trauma.   E. none of the above.
   C. pulse oximetry reading.

_____ 4. If you arrive at your patient's side only moments after the serious trauma event, he may not have lost enough blood to demonstrate the signs of shock.
   A. True
   B. False

_____ 5. Which of the following body regions is examined during the rapid trauma assessment?
   A. head   D. thorax
   B. neck   E. all of the above
   C. pelvis

_____ 6. The "B" of DCAP-BTLS stands for:
   A. burns.   D. bilateral injury.
   B. bumps.   E. bruises.
   C. blemishes.

_____ 7. Which of the following is NOT represented within the DCAP-BTLS mnemonic?
   A. contusions   D. crepitation
   B. abrasions   E. swelling
   C. burns

_____ 8. Scalp wounds tend to bleed heavily because:
   A. there is a lack of a protective vasospasm mechanism.
   B. the hair helps continue the blood loss.
   C. the close proximity of the skull permits blood to flow quickly outward.
   D. direct pressure is difficult to apply.
   E. both A and C.

_____ 9. Subcutaneous emphysema is best described as:
   A. a grating sensation.
   B. air trapped under the skin.
   C. air leaking from the respiratory system.
   D. retraction of the tissues between the ribs.
   E. fluid accumulation just beneath the skin.

_____ 10. Suprasternal and intercostal retractions are caused by:
   A. tension pneumothorax.   D. flail chest.
   B. subcutaneous emphysema.   E. either B or D.
   C. airway obstruction or restriction.

_____ 11. To ensure adequate air exchange for the patient with a flail chest,
          you should:
   A. perform a needle decompression.
   B. assist ventilations with a BVM and oxygen.
   C. apply oxygen only.
   D. perform an endotracheal intubation.
   E. cover the wound with an occlusive dressing.

_____ 12. When assessing the pelvis for possible fracture, you should apply:
   A. anterior pressure on the iliac crests.
   B. lateral pressure on the symphysis pubis.
   C. firm pressure on the lower abdomen.
   D. medial and posterior pressure on the iliac crests.
   E. pressure to move the hips to the flexed position.

_____ 13. Your finding that a patient is able to move a limb but the limb is cool, pale,
          and without a pulse is consistent with:
   A. neurologic compromise.
   B. vascular compromise.
   C. both a vascular and a neurologic compromise.
   D. spinal injury.
   E. peripheral nerve root injury.

_____ 14. The "A" of the SAMPLE history stands for:
   A. alcohol consumption.   D. allergies.
   B. adverse reactions.   E. none of the above.
   C. attitude.

_____ 15. With a patient who has a crushing injury to his index finger received when
          it was caught in a closing door, which form of patient assessment would be
          most reasonable?
   A. the rapid trauma assessment and a quick history
   B. the rapid trauma assessment and a detailed history
   C. a quick history and a physical exam focused on the injury
   D. a detailed patient history and a physical exam focused on the injury
   E. a detailed physical exam

_____ 16. While gathering the history of a chest pain patient, you will likely:
   A. attach a cardiac monitor.   D. start an IV, if appropriate.
   B. administer oxygen.   E. all of the above.
   C. take vital signs.

_____ 17. The pain or discomfort that caused the patient to call you to his side
          is called the:
   A. presenting problem.   D. chief complaint.
   B. differential diagnosis.   E. present illness.
   C. field diagnosis.

_____ 18. A patient statement that "deep breathing makes my chest hurt" represents
          which element of the OPQRST-ASPN mnemonic for investigation
          of the chief complaint?
   A. O   D. S
   B. P   E. PN
   C. R

©2009 Pearson Education, Inc.
Paramedic Care: Principles & Practice, Vol. 2, 3rd. Ed.

_____ 19. The jugular veins in a patient with normal cardiovascular function remain full or distended up to which of the following degrees of patient tilt?
A. 15°
B. 30°
C. 45°
D. 60°
E. 90°

_____ 20. If you hear bilateral crackles on inspiration when auscultating a patient's chest, you should suspect:
A. congestive heart failure.
B. bronchospasm.
C. asthma.
D. chronic obstructive pulmonary disease.
E. all of the above.

_____ 21. In a patient who displays hyperresonance to percussion, you should suspect:
A. pleural effusion.
B. pulmonary edema.
C. pneumonia.
D. emphysema.
E. none of the above.

_____ 22. Examine a patient for unusual pulsation of the descending aorta:
A. just right of the umbilicus.
B. just left of the umbilicus.
C. along a line from the umbilicus to the middle symphysis pubis.
D. just beneath the zyphoid process.
E. anywhere in the abdomen.

_____ 23. Accumulation of fluid within the abdominal cavity is common in patients with:
A. hypovolemia.
B. aortic aneurysm.
C. emphysema.
D. gastric ulcer disease.
E. cirrhosis of the liver.

_____ 24. A patient in whom unequal pupils are a normal condition displays:
A. Cullen's sign.
B. anisocoria.
C. consensual response.
D. accommodation.
E. Bell's palsy.

_____ 25. Vital signs provide the assessing paramedic with:
A. a window into what is happening with the patient.
B. an objective capsule of the patient's clinical status.
C. possible indications of severe illness.
D. possible indications of the need to intervene.
E. all of the above.

_____ 26. A pulse oximetry reading of 88 percent would indicate the need for:
A. aggressive airway and ventilatory care.
B. only the administration of blow-by oxygen.
C. only some repositioning of the patient's head.
D. no care at this point.
E. careful monitoring of the patient for further deterioration.

_____ 27. The type of patient most likely to receive the most comprehensive assessment is:
A. the severe trauma patient.
B. the minor trauma patient.
C. the responsive medical patient.
D. the unresponsive medical patient.
E. both A and D.

_____ 28. Paramedics employ the complete detailed physical assessment at the scene:
A. rarely.
B. occasionally.
C. frequently.
D. rarely in trauma patients, frequently in medical patients.
E. frequently in trauma patients, rarely in medical patients.

_____ **29.** Reflexes not likely to be tested during the detailed physical exam are the:

    A. clavicular.

    B. biceps.

    C. triceps.

    D. Achilles.

    E. abdominal plantar.

_____ **30.** Serial ongoing assessments will facilitate:

    A. reassessment of the patient.

    B. revision of the field diagnosis.

    C. changes in the management plan.

    D. documentation of the effects of interventions.

    E. all of the above.

Special Project

Cranial Nerve Testing—Personal Benchmarking

One complicated element of the physical assessment is the evaluation of the 12 cranial nerves. You must learn not only the skill itself but also how to perform it quickly in the field, often under adverse conditions. To help with this process, attempt to evaluate the cranial nerves on yourself. This can aid you in remembering both the steps of the process and the normal and expected responses. This exercise can also help you maintain this skill during your career as a paramedic. Please review text pages 226 to 227.

    To perform this examination, you will need a retractable ballpoint pen, a penlight, some cotton swabs, a large full-length mirror, some cologne or perfume, and, for some tests, a partner. Practice this exam a few times; then repeat it a day or so later until it becomes a natural procedure. Doing so will help you when called upon to check the cranial nerves in class or on a patient.

    I Olfactory (smell): Close your eyes and one nostril and then sense for various odors. Use a perfume, a cologne, or another nonirritating agent. You should be able to recognize various smells through each nostril. _(This check is not often performed in the field.)_

    II Optic (visual acuity, peripheral vision): Evaluate each eye for visual acuity by testing gross image recognition at about 20 feet. Look for the smallest item you can discern. _Use your visual acuity (20/20, 20/40, or whatever) as a benchmark against which to gauge your patient's visual acuity (his eyesight is better, the same, or worse)._ Then extend your arms, move them backward, behind your line of view, and wiggle your fingers. While looking straight ahead, bring the fingers forward until they just come into view. The angle made between your fingers and the tip of your nose is the angle of your peripheral vision, usually about 180 degrees. _Perform this test on a patient by placing yourself face to face with him, extending an arm on each side of his head behind his ears, then bringing your hands slowly forward while wiggling your fingers. Measure the point at which he first notices your fingers._

    III Oculomotor (pupillary responsiveness): _This response should be tested on a partner because it is hard to watch the motions of your own eyes._ Inspect the size, shape, and equality of the pupils. A slight inequality may be normal. With the room otherwise dark, shine a penlight obliquely toward the pupil. The light should cause both the affected and opposite pupil to constrict briskly (consensual response). Then check for near response. Have your partner follow your finger as you move it toward his nose. Watch for the eyes to converge and the pupils to constrict.

    III Oculomotor, IV Trochlear, and VI Abducens (eye muscle control): _Again, this response should be tested on a partner or someone else, because you cannot watch your eye motion in the mirror and follow your finger at the same time._ Test extraocular movement (EOM) by having your partner follow the tip of your finger while you trace an "H" in front of each eye. As you move your finger, watch the eye and halt lateral motion when the eye stops moving with the finger. Then move the finger up and down while continuing to watch the pupil. Ensure that the eyes move together. In the field, any restriction of motion should suggest muscle paralysis or possibly entrapment by an orbital fracture.

©2009 Pearson Education, Inc.
Paramedic Care: Principles & Practice, Vol. 2, 3rd. Ed.

V Trigeminal (facial muscles and sensation): Test the trigeminal nerve function by clenching your teeth and palpating the muscle tone. For sensory testing, check for bilateral touch sensation on the forehead, cheek, and chin using a sharp object (such as the tip of a ballpoint pen with the ball retracted) and a dull object (such as a cotton ball). Last, touch the cornea of the eyes with a few strands of the fibers of a cotton ball and expect an immediate blink.

VII Facial (facial features and eyelids): Closely observe your facial features for general shape and symmetry. Then raise your eyebrows, frown, show your upper and lower teeth, smile, and then puff out your cheeks. Close your eyes tightly and attempt to open them with finger pressure. Any unilateral strength, facial droop, or asymmetrical movement may be a result of nerve injury (possibly Bell's palsy).

VIII Acoustic (hearing and balance): Occlude one ear with a finger and lightly tap the fingers of the opposite hand near the open auditory canal. Hearing should be clear and bilaterally equal. *For a patient, whisper something softly in the nonoccluded ear and ask him to repeat it.* Then check balance by closing your eyes for 5 or 10 seconds and noticing your position in the mirror after you open them. You should still be standing straight, not wavering, and you should not experience vertigo. *The patient should not move around more than when his eyes are open.*

IX Glossopharyngeal and X Vagus (speech and tongue control): Listen carefully to your voice and articulation of words while looking in the mirror. Your voice should not be hoarse (vocal cord problem) or nasal in tone (palate problem), and it should be clear and distinct. Say "aaahhh" and watch through the open mouth. The uvula and palate should rise symmetrically while the posterior pharynx moves medially.

XI Accessory (shoulder and neck muscles): Examine the positioning of the shoulder (trapezius) and neck (sternocleidomastoid) muscles for symmetry at rest. Raise each shoulder against resistance from the opposite hand *(have a patient raise both simultaneously)*. Then turn your head against resistance (using your hands) to the left, then right. Any unilateral weakness suggests nerve injury.

XII Hypoglossal (tongue): Stick out your tongue and watch for midline projection. It should remain straight and not deviate. Then move your tongue from side to side. Again, the motions should be symmetrical. *Any deviation is usually away from the affected side.*

4

Clinical Decision Making

Review of Chapter Objectives

After reading this chapter, you should be able to:

1. **Compare the factors influencing medical care in the out-of-hospital environment to other medical settings.** **p. 246**

   Most health care providers function in very controlled and supportive environments. The paramedic carries out the skills of other health care providers, but he often does so in hostile and adverse conditions. Paramedics perform assessments, form field diagnoses, and devise and employ patient management plans at the scenes of emergencies in spite of poor weather, limited ambient light, limited diagnostic equipment, and few support personnel. The paramedic also must perform these skills under extreme constraints of time and often without on-scene consultation and supervision.

2. **Differentiate between critical life-threatening, potentially life-threatening, and nonlife-threatening patient presentations.** **pp. 249–250**

   Critical life-threatening presentations include major multi-system trauma, devastating single system trauma, end-stage disease presentations, and acute presentations of chronic disease. These patients may present with airway, breathing, neurologic, or circulatory (shock) problems and demand aggressive resuscitation.

   Potential life-threatening presentations include serious multi-system trauma and multiple disease etiologies. Patient presentation generally includes moderate to serious distress. The care required is sometimes invasive but generally supportive.

   Nonlife-threatening presentations are isolated and uncomplicated minor injuries or illness. The patient is stable without serious signs or symptoms or the need for aggressive intervention.

3. **Evaluate the benefits and shortfalls of protocols, standing orders, and patient care algorithms.** **p. 250**

   Protocols are written guidelines identifying the specific management of various medical and trauma patient problems. They may also be developed for special situations, such as physician-on-the-scene, radio failure, and termination of resuscitation. They provide a standard care approach for patients with classical presentations. They do not apply to all patients or to patients who present with multiple problems and should not be adhered to so rigidly as to limit performance in unusual circumstances.

   Standing orders are protocols that a paramedic can perform before direct on-line communication with a medical direction physician. They speed emergency care but may not address the atypical patient.

Patient care algorithms are flow charts with lines, arrows, and boxes that outline appropriate care measures based on patient presentation or response to care. They are generally useful guides and encourage uniform patient care, but, again, they do not adequately address the atypical patient.

4. **Define the components, stages, and sequences of the critical thinking process for paramedics.** pp. 250–258

Components of critical thinking include those discussed in the following section.

Knowledge and Abilities

Knowledge and abilities are the first component of critical thinking. Your knowledge of prehospital emergency care is the basis for your decisions in the field. This knowledge comes from your classroom, clinical, and field experience. It is used to sort out your patient's presentation to determine the likely cause of the problem and to select the appropriate care skills. Your abilities are the technical skills you employ to assess or care for a patient.

Useful Thinking Styles

- **Reflective vs. impulsive situation analysis.** "Reflective analysis" refers to taking time to deliberately and analytically contemplate possible patient care, as might occur with an unknown medical illness. "Impulsive analysis" refers to the immediate response that the paramedic must provide in a life-threatening situation, as might be required with decompensating shock or cardiac arrest.
- **Divergent vs. convergent data processing.** Divergent data processing considers all aspects of a situation before arriving at a solution and is most useful with complex situations. Convergent data processing focuses narrowly on the most important aspects of a situation and is best suited for uncomplicated situations that require little reflection.
- **Anticipatory vs. reactive decision making.** With anticipatory decision making, you respond to what you think may happen to your patient. With reactive decision making, you provide a care modality once the patient presents with a symptom.

Thinking under Pressure

Thinking under pressure is a difficult but frequent challenge of prehospital emergency medicine. The "fight or flight" response may diminish your ability to think critically to such an extent that you are able to respond only at the pseudo-instinctive level, with preplanned and practiced responses (such as the mental checklist) that are performed almost without thought. One example of a mental checklist includes the following steps:

1. *Scan the situation* by standing back and looking for subtle clues to the patient's complaint or problem.

2. *Stop and think* of both the possible benefits and the side effects of each of your care interventions.

3. *Decide and act* by executing your chosen care plan with confidence and authority.

4. *Maintain control* of the scene, patient care, and your own emotions, even under the stress of a chaotic scene.

5. *Reevaluate* your patient's signs and symptoms and your associated care plan and make changes as the situation changes.

5. **Apply the fundamental elements of critical thinking for paramedics.** pp. 256–258

Form a concept. Gather enough information from your first view of the patient and scene size-up to form a general impression of the patient's condition and the likely cause.

Interpret the data. Perform the patient assessment and analyze the results in light of your previous assessment and care experience. Form a field diagnosis.

Apply the principles. With the field diagnosis in mind, devise a management plan to care for the patient according to your protocols, standing orders, and patient care algorithms.

©2009 Pearson Education, Inc.
Paramedic Care: Principles & Practice, Vol. 2, 3rd. Ed.

Evaluate. Through frequent ongoing assessments, reassess the patient's condition and the effects of your interventions.

Reflect. After the call, critique your call with the emergency department staff and your crew to determine what steps might be improved and add this call to your experience base.

6. Describe the effects of the "fight or flight" response and its positive and negative effects on a paramedic's decision making. p. 255

The "fight or flight" response is the intense activation of the sympathetic branch of the autonomic nervous system. Secretion of the system's major hormone, epinephrine, causes an increase in heart rate and cardiac output. It raises respiratory rate and volume, directs blood to the skeletal muscles, dilates the pupils (for distant vision), and increases hearing perception. However, the increased epinephrine may diminish critical thinking ability and concentration, impairing your ability to perform well in an emergency unless you raise your assessment and care skills to a pseudo-instinctive level, at which point acting under the pressure of an emergency becomes second nature.

7. Summarize the "six *R*s" of putting it all together. p. 258

Read the patient. Observe, palpate, auscultate, smell, and listen to the patient for signs and symptoms. Ensure the ABCs and obtain a set of vital signs.

Read the scene. Observe the scene or general environment for clues to the mechanism of injury or nature of the illness.

React. Address the priorities of care from the ABCs to other critical, then serious, then minor problems and care priorities.

Reevaluate. Conduct frequent ongoing assessments to identify any changes caused either by the disease or by your interventions.

Revise the management plan. Based on the ongoing assessments, revise your management plan to best serve your patient's changing condition.

Review performance. At the end of every response, critique the performance of your crew and identify ways to improve future responses.

8. Given several preprogrammed and moulaged trauma and medical patients, demonstrate clinical decision making. pp. 248–258

With your classroom, clinical, and field experience, you will assess and develop a management plan for the real and simulated patients you attend. Use the information presented in this text chapter, the information on clinical decision making presented by your instructors, and the guidance given by your clinical and field preceptors to develop good clinical decision-making skills. Continue to refine these skills once your training ends and you begin your career as a paramedic.

Case Study Review

Reread the case study on page 247 in Paramedic Care: Patient Assessment *and then read the following discussion.*

This case study describes a typical trauma patient. The paramedic's primary survey suggests serious impact, but the patient at first demonstrates no signs or symptoms of serious internal injury. As assessment, care, and transport proceed, however, the patient deteriorates, requiring the paramedic to employ critical clinical decision-making skills.

Sue responds to a routine trauma call. After performing a primary survey and a rapid trauma assessment, Sue decides that the patient does not meet the criteria for rapid transport to a trauma center. Sue's rapid trauma assessment suggests that Marcie has experienced only minor facial trauma and the signs and symptoms support that determination. The only point of possible concern is Marcie's inability to remember what happened. However, her hemodynamic status and vital signs support the field diagnosis of minor facial injuries. Her patient acuity is determined to be nonlife-threatening. Sue decides the closest community hospital is a good choice to ensure quick care for Marcie's injuries and cancels the county medevac helicopter.

En route to the community hospital, Sue performs an ongoing assessment (every 15 minutes for a minor injury patient). She discovers that Marcie is showing some signs of a CNS deficit. This causes Sue to reevaluate her original patient acuity and field diagnosis. The degeneration of Marcie's level of responsiveness alarms Sue. Through divergent thinking, looking for other causes of Marcie's presentation, she changes the patient acuity to life-threatening and her field diagnosis to increasing intracranial pressure. She will no doubt now monitor Marcie every 5 minutes and focus her attention on the signs of increasing intracranial pressure, diminishing level of consciousness and orientation, slowing pulse rate, and rising systolic blood pressure. If oxygen has not already been applied, Sue administers it; the urgency of transport increases, and the destination is changed to a trauma center.

Because Sue carefully monitored her patient and employed good critical decision-making skills, Marcie did not go to a community hospital. If she had, she likely would have been stabilized and then transported to a trauma or neuro-center, delaying her time to critical surgery. Such ongoing monitoring of a patient, along with the anticipation of possible responses, will help you provide the best care possible for your patients. As this call ends, Sue and her crew will critique their actions and search for ways to improve the care they give patients with similar presentations.

Content Self-Evaluation

MULTIPLE CHOICE

_____ 1. Which of the following terms best describes the first paramedics of the 1970s?
A. field technicians
B. prehospital emergency care practitioners
C. orderlies
D. field attendants
E. field aides

_____ 2. The term describing the severity of a patient's condition is:
A. multiparity.
B. epiphysis.
C. tonicity.
D. acuity.
E. declivity.

_____ 3. The paramedic's final determination of the patient's most likely primary problem is known as the:
A. field diagnosis.
B. differential field diagnosis.
C. chief complaint.
D. improvisation.
E. standing order.

_____ 4. Which of the following is NOT a level of patient acuity?
A. life-threatening condition
B. nonlife-threatening condition
C. potential nonlife-threatening condition
D. potential life-threatening condition
E. both A and B

_____ 5. Which patient acuity level presents the greatest challenge to the paramedic's critical thinking skills?
A. life-threatening condition
B. nonlife-threatening condition
C. potential nonlife-threatening condition
D. potential life-threatening condition
E. B and C equally

©2009 Pearson Education, Inc.
Paramedic Care: Principles & Practice, Vol. 2, 3rd. Ed.

_____ 6. Which of the following represents a flow chart of patient care procedures?
  A. protocol
  B. standing order
  C. algorithm
  D. special care enhancement
  E. proviso

_____ 7. A policy of administering nitroglycerin to a cardiac chest pain patient is an example of a(n):
  A. protocol.
  B. standing order.
  C. algorithm.
  D. special care enhancement.
  E. proviso.

_____ 8. A policy by which nitroglycerin can be administered to a cardiac chest pain patient without a physician's order is an example of a(n):
  A. protocol.
  B. standing order.
  C. algorithm.
  D. special enhancement.
  E. proviso.

_____ 9. The major disadvantage to the use of protocols and standing orders is that they:
  A. apply only to atypical patients.
  B. often do not permit the paramedic to adapt to a patient's unique presentation.
  C. only cover multiple disease etiologies.
  D. address only patients with vague presentations.
  E. none of the above.

_____ 10. When a particular protocol does not seem to fit the patient presentation, you should contact the medical direction physician for advice and direction regarding your patient's care.
  A. True
  B. False

_____ 11. The data-processing style that focuses on the most important aspect of a critical situation is:
  A. reflective.
  B. impulsive.
  C. divergent.
  D. convergent.
  E. anticipatory.

_____ 12. The style of situation analysis that causes you to respond instinctively to a situation rather than to think about it is:
  A. reflective.
  B. impulsive.
  C. divergent.
  D. convergent.
  E. anticipatory.

_____ 13. One way to remain in control in otherwise extremely stressful situations is to learn to perform technical skills at a pseudo-instinctive level.
  A. True
  B. False

_____ 14. Which of the following is NOT a step in the critical decision-making process?
  A. forming a concept
  B. interpreting the data
  C. applying the principles
  D. evaluating the result
  E. evaluating the interventions

_____ 15. Which of the following is NOT an element of the six "Rs" of critical decision making?
  A. reading the scene
  B. researching the management plan
  C. reacting
  D. reading the patient
  E. reevaluating

MATCHING

Write the letter of the step in the critical decision-making process in the space provided next to the emergency response action appropriate for that step.

_____ 16. Field diagnosis

_____ 17. Provide ongoing assessment.

_____ 18. Perform the focused physical exam.

_____ 19. Pulse oximetry

_____ 20. Follow standing orders.

_____ 21. Differential diagnosis

_____ 22. Assess MS-ABCs.

_____ 23. Employ protocols.

_____ 24. Determine the initial vital signs.

_____ 25. Determine if treatment is improving the patient's condition.

A. Form a concept.

B. Interpret the data.

C. Apply the principles.

D. Evaluate.

E. Reflect.

©2009 Pearson Education, Inc.
Paramedic Care: Principles & Practice, Vol. 2, 3rd. Ed.

Communications

Review of Chapter Objectives

After reading this chapter, you should be able to:

1. Identify the role and importance of verbal, written, and electronic communications in the provision of EMS.   **pp. 266–275**

EMS is a team endeavor that requires effective communications among the various participants in the response and patient care. This communication is between you and the emergency dispatcher; the patient; the patient's family; bystanders; other emergency response personnel, such as police, fire, and rescue personnel; health care professionals from physicians' offices, clinics, and emergency departments; and the medical direction physician. These communications, be they oral, written, or electronic, establish the key links that ensure the best patient outcome.

2. Describe the phases of communications necessary to complete a typical EMS response.

Detection and Citizen Access   **pp. 269–275**

This marks the initial entry point into the emergency service system at which a party identifies that an emergency exists and then requests EMS assistance through a universal entry number, such as 911, or some other mechanism.

Call Taking   **p. 273**

This is the stage of EMS response in which a call taker questions the caller about the reported emergency to identify its exact location, to determine the nature of the call, and to initiate an appropriate response.

Emergency Response   **p. 273**

This phase includes the activities occurring from the moment a dispatcher requests a response by an EMS unit until the call concludes with the unit back in service. It includes various radio, face-to-face, and written communications among the dispatcher, emergency response crews, patient, family and bystanders, and health care professionals, including the medical direction physician.

Prearrival Instructions   **pp. 273–274**

These are a series of predetermined, medically approved instructions the dispatcher gives the caller to help the caller provide some patient support until EMS personnel arrive.

Call Coordination and Incident Recording   **pp. 274–275**

The terms "call coordination" and "incident recording" refer to the interactions between the dispatcher and the responding units that ensure an efficient and appropriate response. Call coordinating, for example, might involve changing the mode of response and the number and type of responding units. "Incident recording" refers to the logging of times associated with various response activities and the tape recording of communications associated with the call.

Discussion with the Medical Direction Physician   p. 275

This is the opportunity for the care provider to describe the patient he is caring for and to obtain approval from the medical direction physician to initiate invasive or advanced life support procedures. Communication with medical direction also permits the emergency department to prepare for the patient's arrival.

Transfer Communications   p. 275

Transfer communications are those that occur between the first responder and the paramedic or as the patient is delivered to the emergency department. They are intended to communicate the results of the assessment, the care given, and the patient's response to care before the arrival of the paramedic or arrival at the emergency department.

3. **List factors that impede and enhance effective verbal and written communications.** pp. 265–268

The factors affecting effective verbal or written communications are either semantic (dealing with the meaning of words) or technical (hardware).

In the area of semantics, the use of standard codes and plain English in verbal communications enhances good and clear communications, while the use of nonstandard codes and jargon may confuse it. The same holds true for written communication. Nonstandard abbreviations and subjective, sloppy, incomplete, or illegible documentation leads to confusion and miscommunication. Complete, objective, legible, and efficient documentation leads to an efficient transfer of information. A well-designed prehospital care report makes written communication easier.

In the technical area, a well-designed and maintained radio or phone communications system will go a long way in ensuring good and dependable communications. Improperly maintained or operated radios will, on the other hand, likely provide only intermittent and poor-quality communication.

4. **Explain the value of data collection during an EMS response.** p. 267

The written call report is a record that includes the patient's name and address, the scene location, the agency responding, the crew on board, and the times associated with response, arrival, and transport to a care facility. It also contains the results of the assessment and care of the patient. This administrative information can be used to bill for services and improve EMS system efficiency, can be used by quality assurance/improvement committees to improve system performance, and can be used by educators and researchers to identify what the system is doing and the effects of its interventions. Finally, the call report becomes a legal record of the incident and the EMS care provided or offered.

5. **Recognize the legal status of verbal, written, and electronic communications related to an EMS response.** pp. 266–268

The legal guidelines that apply to verbal and written communications in EMS also apply to electronic communications. The information in these communications is considered confidential and must be released only in approved circumstances. The reports must be objective and not demean, libel, or slander another person. Any such action is accountable in a court of law.

6. **Identify current and new technology used to collect and exchange patient and/or scene information electronically.** pp. 276–280

Cellular phones provide duplex communications directly from the patient's side to the emergency department. These lightweight and versatile devices enhance EMS-to-physician communications and permit excellent ECG transmission. The only disadvantages to cell phones are user fees and unreliability at peak times.

Another electronic aid to dispatch is the facsimile, or fax, machine. It permits dispatch to send hard copy to the responding unit's station, ensuring that elements of the address and nature of the dispatch are communicated accurately.

©2009 Pearson Education, Inc.
Paramedic Care: Principles & Practice, Vol. 2, 3rd. Ed.

Computers are also increasing the efficiency of the dispatch system by recording times and system action in real time and making data recovery and research much easier.

Other new technologies that may affect prehospital care include the electronic touch pad, which allows rapid recording of patient information; the handheld computer, which uses a pen-based system to log patient information and times associated with the emergency response and care; and electronic transmission of diagnostic information (including pulse oximetry, 12-lead ECG, blood glucose, and capnography monitoring) directly to the emergency department, which may change the degree and number of field interventions permitted. In the future, voice recognition software may make real-time narrative recording of patient evaluation and interventions at the emergency scene and during transport a reality.

7. Identify the various components of the EMS communications system and describe their function and use. pp. 269–275

The emergency medical dispatcher (EMD) is the person who takes the call for assistance, dispatches the appropriate units, monitors the call's progress, and ensures that the pertinent response data are recorded. The EMD may guide the caller through initial emergency care using prearrival instructions.

The patient, his family, and bystanders are responsible for detecting the emergency, accessing the emergency response system, and relaying information about the cause and nature of the emergency to EMS system personnel. These individuals are not trained in emergency medical communication, and therefore the responsibility of ensuring good communications falls on the members of the EMS system.

Personnel from other responding agencies, such as the police, fire service, rescue, and other ambulance services, also provide information important to ensuring proper EMS response, and their input must be taken into account for scene coordination and optimum utilization of resources.

Health care professionals (aides, nurses, physician assistants, nurse practitioners, and physicians) at clinics, physicians' offices, and emergency departments are important people in the EMS system. They can provide invaluable information about the patient and the care he has had or should receive.

Finally, the medical director and medical direction physicians are significant resources for the prehospital emergency care provider. They are the individuals who extend their licenses to paramedics, thereby permitting them to practice prehospital care. These physicians also represent a body of knowledge of emergency medicine that may be tapped while paramedics are at the scene, en route with a patient, or at the emergency department for guidance regarding patient care.

8. Identify and differentiate among the following communications systems.

Simplex p. 276
The simplex system is a radio or communication system that uses only one frequency and allows only one unit to transmit at a time. With this type of communication, one party must wait until the speaking party completes his message before beginning to speak.

Duplex p. 276
The radio or communication system that uses two frequencies for each channel, thus permitting two units to transmit and listen at the same time, is the duplex system. This is similar to telephone communication, in which one party can interrupt the other.

Multiplex p. 277
Multiplex is a duplex system with an additional capability of transmitting data, such as an ECG strip, simultaneously with voice.

Trunked p. 277
These are computer-controlled systems that pool all radio frequencies and assign transmissions to unused frequencies to ensure the most efficient use of available communications channels.

Digital communications

pp. 277–278

These systems translate analog sounds into digital code for transmissions that are less prone to interference and are more compact than analog (normal voice) communications. This type of a system can be enhanced with devices such as the mobile data terminal, which displays information such as street addresses, and can prompt the responder to send information such as "arrived."

Cellular telephone

p. 278

Cellular telephones are part of a multiplex radio-telephone system tied to a computer that uses radio towers to transmit signals in regions called cells. The technology is inexpensive but can accrue substantial monthly charges; the transmissions may be interrupted by certain geographic features; and heavy use at peak times may limit access to the system.

Facsimile

p. 278

Facsimile machines transmit and receive printed information through telephone or wireless communication systems. Such a machine might give a responding unit a printout of the nature and street address of the call or detailed medical information about it.

Computer

p. 279

The use of computers in EMS is expanding rapidly. They are already helping analyze data for review of calls and dispatches. Portable input devices, such as the touch pad and handheld computer, are being developed to permit recording of emergency response events in the field. In the future, paramedics may use computers with voice recognition software to complete prehospital care reports without paper.

9. **Describe the functions and responsibilities of the Federal Communications Commission.**

p. 282

The Federal Communications Commission (FCC) controls and regulates all nongovernmental communications in the United States. It assigns broadcast frequencies and has set aside several frequencies within each radio bandwidth for EMS. The commission also establishes technical standards for radio equipment, licenses and regulates people who repair radios, monitors frequencies for appropriate usage, and checks base stations and dispatch centers for appropriate licenses and records.

10. **Describe the role of emergency medical dispatch and the importance of prearrival instructions in a typical EMS response.**

pp. 269–224

The emergency medical dispatcher (EMD) is the first person in the EMS system who communicates with the scene and possibly the patient. He begins and coordinates the EMS response and communications and ensures that data regarding the call are recorded. He also provides prearrival instructions to callers—for example, how to perform mouth-to-mouth artificial ventilation on an apneic patient—so that emergency care can begin as early as possible, thus helping maintain the victim until trained prehospital personnel can arrive.

11. **List appropriate caller information gathered by the emergency medical dispatcher.**

pp. 269–273

The information the EMD gathers to determine the response priority and that is then communicated to the appropriate responding EMS service includes

- Caller's name
- Call-back number
- Location or address of the event
- Nature of the call
- Any additional information necessary to prioritize the call

©2009 Pearson Education, Inc.
Paramedic Care: Principles & Practice, Vol. 2, 3rd. Ed.

12. Describe the structure and importance of verbal patient information communication to the hospital and medical direction. pp. 280–281

The verbal patient report to hospital personnel and the medical direction physician is essential to ensure the efficient transfer and continuity of care. It consists of the following:

- Information identifying the care provider and level of training
- Patient identification information (name, age, sex, and so on)
- Subjective patient data (for example, chief complaint, additional symptoms, past history)
- Objective patient data (vital signs, pulse oximetry readings, and so on)
- Plan for care of the patient

For the trauma patient, the information and order of presentation is the same, although the subjective and objective information is modified to include mechanism of injury and suspected injuries.

13. Diagram a basic communications system. pp. 266–267

Basic communication is the process of exchanging information between individuals. A model for a communications system should start with an idea, followed by encoding that idea into useful language, sending the encoded message via a medium (direct voice, radio, or written medium), having another person receive and decode the message, and, ultimately, receiving feedback from the original message.

14. Given several narrative patient scenarios, organize a verbal radio report for electronic transmission to medical direction. pp. 264–282

During your classroom, clinical, and field training, you will communicate with various elements of the EMS system, including dispatchers, patients, family members, bystanders, other EMS and scene personnel, and health care professionals, including medical direction physicians. Use the information presented in this text chapter, the information on communication presented by your instructors, and the guidance given by your clinical and field preceptors to develop good communication skills. Continue to refine these skills once your training ends and you begin your career as a paramedic.

Case Study Review

Reread the case study on pages 263 and 264 in Paramedic Care: Patient Assessment *and then read the following discussion.*

This case study discusses an emergency call and the elements of communications—specifically, the radio communications between the paramedic and medical direction.

This case study identifies some of the common and critical elements of communication essential to the emergency response. First, someone needs to recognize an emergency exists (detection), and then he must contact the emergency response system (access). The dispatcher must then receive the call (call taking), determine its nature and seriousness, and dispatch the appropriate resources to deal with the problem (emergency response). The dispatcher determines the priority of the call by asking the caller a series of medically approved questions. The dispatcher, in addition, provides the caller with basic, approved first-aid steps to perform (prearrival instructions) until EMS reaches the scene to supply more comprehensive care. The dispatcher also coordinates the responses of any fire, police, rescue, or other service units needed to the scene (call coordination). The dispatch center records the pertinent information and times associated with the call for further review by the system administrator, the medical director, the quality improvement committee, researchers, or attorneys (incident recording).

Once at the scene and actively involved in patient care, the care providers contact medical direction to communicate the patient's condition and the care they have begun. This communication paints a clear picture of the patient they are treating. It may stimulate questions from the physician regarding the findings and patient care and may elicit orders for invasive actions, such as starting an IV line or administering medications. When the paramedic communicates with medical direction regarding orders for invasive actions, he uses the echo procedure, repeating back the physician's orders word for word to ensure that both parties understand what is to be done.

The communications between the paramedics and medical direction also enable the emergency department staff to prepare for the arrival of the patient (transfer communications). In this case, the patient's condition is critical and time is of the essence. When the patient arrives, the hospital is ready for immediate surgery. While in this case prehospital and hospital care do not result in patient survival, support of the patient's vital signs provides organs that are used to prolong other lives.

Another factor to consider in this case study is the hardware necessary to the EMS response. The cellular phone makes communications from a bystander at the accident site possible, and the system is alerted quickly to the patient's plight. A system status management and priority dispatch system ensures ambulances are close to the areas where response is needed and allows for coordinated responses. It also ensures that red lights and sirens are used only for true emergencies. The Enhanced 911 system uses a computer to determine the quickest route to the scene and provides the responding ambulance electronically with a printout of all the pertinent information needed to respond without taking the dispatcher away from the caller. The paramedics probably send an ECG to Dr. Doyle while they speak (multiplex), and Dr. Doyle can interrupt them as they deliver their report to ask questions (duplex). This hardware and a coordinated system of communication provide the best response and care for the patients of this EMS system.

Content Self-Evaluation

MULTIPLE CHOICE

_____ 1. Essential participants in communications within the EMS system include:
   A. the emergency medical dispatcher.
   B. the patient, his family, or bystanders.
   C. other responders, including police, fire, and other ambulance personnel.
   D. health care providers, including nurses, physicians, and medical direction physicians.
   E. all of the above.

_____ 2. In general, the use of codes decreases the radio time and increases the recipient's understanding of the message, which has led many EMS systems to adopt extensive use of codes for their communications.
   A. True
   B. False

_____ 3. A radio band is a:
   A. series of radios that communicate with one another.
   B. pair of radio frequencies used for multiplexing.
   C. range of radio frequencies.
   D. pair of radio frequencies used for duplexing.
   E. none of the above.

_____ 4. Use of proper terminology in both written and verbal communications will:
   A. decrease the length of communications.
   B. increase the accuracy of communications.
   C. increase the clarity of communications.
   D. reduce the ambiguity in communications.
   E. all of the above.

©2009 Pearson Education, Inc.
Paramedic Care: Principles & Practice, Vol. 2, 3rd. Ed.

_____ 5. Features of the Enhanced 911 center include all of the following EXCEPT:
   A. display of the caller's location.
   B. display of the caller's phone number.
   C. immediate call-back ability.
   D. a system of physician/ambulance interface.
   E. both B and C.

_____ 6. The answering center for emergency calls, which then transfers them to the appropriate agency for dispatch, is the:
   A. Enhanced 911 center.
   B. PSAP.
   C. GPS.
   D. emergency routing center.
   E. none of the above.

_____ 7. Most current wireless phones do not provide the PSAP with the phone's location and call-back number.
   A. True
   B. False

_____ 8. Which system may identify the exact location of a wireless phone?
   A. geographic triangulation
   B. landline induction
   C. global positioning system
   D. either A or C
   E. none of the above

_____ 9. Terrestrial-based triangulation of a wireless phone's location is dependent on which of the following?
   A. signal strength
   B. height of the wireless phone antenna
   C. three towers receiving the signal
   D. the proximity of the PSAP
   E. both A and C

_____ 10. The Enhanced 911 center may soon be notified of a vehicle collision, the forces involved, and its location through which of the following technological enhancements?
   A. ANI
   B. ALI
   C. ACN
   D. PSAP
   E. none of the above

_____ 11. In the future, which of the following may be communicated to the dispatch center from a vehicle involved in a collision?
   A. the exact location of the incident
   B. a change in velocity of the collision
   C. the vehicle identification number
   D. the crash worthiness rating of the vehicle involved
   E. all of the above

_____ 12. The system that uses standardized caller questioning to determine the level and type of response is:
   A. priority dispatching.
   B. system status management.
   C. enhanced emergency medical dispatch.
   D. prearrival instructions packaging.
   E. dispatch triage.

_____ 13. The role of the modern-day emergency medical dispatcher includes:
  A. priority dispatching.
  B. prearrival instructions.
  C. call coordinating.
  D. incident recording.
  E. all of the above.

_____ 14. The report that occurs as you transfer patient responsibilities to the emergency department staff must include:
  A. chief complaint.
  B. assessment findings.
  C. care rendered.
  D. results of care.
  E. all of the above.

_____ 15. A radio system that transmits and receives on the same frequency is called:
  A. simplex.
  B. duplex.
  C. triplex.
  D. multiplex.
  E. none of the above.

_____ 16. Which radio transmission design permits the receiver to interrupt the caller while the caller is talking?
  A. simplex
  B. duplex
  C. multiplex
  D. trunking
  E. none of the above

_____ 17. The radio system that uses a computer to determine and assign available frequencies is called:
  A. simplex.
  B. duplex.
  C. multiplex.
  D. trunking.
  E. none of the above.

_____ 18. Advantages of cellular communications in EMS include all of the following EXCEPT:
  A. duplex capability.
  B. direct physician/patient communication.
  C. ability to handle an unlimited number of calls.
  D. reduced on-line times.
  E. transmission of better ECG signals.

_____ 19. One of the paramedic's most important skills is gathering essential patient information, organizing it, and communicating it to the medical direction physician.
  A. True
  B. False

_____ 20. A standard format for transmitting patient information ensures all of the following EXCEPT:
  A. communication efficiency.
  B. physician assimilation of patient condition information.
  C. completeness of medical information.
  D. easier use of multiplex signals.
  E. both A and C.

©2009 Pearson Education, Inc.
Paramedic Care: Principles & Practice, Vol. 2, 3rd. Ed.

_____ 21. All of the following are appropriate for good EMS communications EXCEPT:
   A. speaking close to the microphone.
   B. speaking across or directly into the microphone.
   C. talking in a normal tone of voice.
   D. speaking without emotion.
   E. taking time to explain everything in detail.

_____ 22. It is important to press the microphone button for 1 second before speaking.
   A. True
   B. False

_____ 23. If the portable radio you are using is unable to transmit well from your location, attempt to:
   A. move to higher ground.
   B. touch the antenna to something metal.
   C. move toward a window or away from structural steel.
   D. both A and C.
   E. none of the above.

_____ 24. The major difference between the medical and trauma patient reports is that the trauma format provides a description of the mechanism of injury and identifies suspected injuries.
   A. True
   B. False

_____ 25. The Federal Communications Commission is responsible for all of the following EXCEPT:
   A. assigning and licensing radio frequencies.
   B. establishing technical standards for radio equipment.
   C. ensuring the proper use of medical terminology in radio communications.
   D. monitoring radio frequencies for proper use.
   E. spot checking radio base stations for proper licensing and records.

Special Project

Documentation: Radio Report/Prehospital Care Report

The authoring of both the radio message to the receiving hospital and the written run report are two of the most important tasks you will perform as a paramedic. Read the following paragraphs, compose a radio message, and complete the run report for this call.

The Call

At 1515 hours, your ambulance, Unit 89, is paged out to an unconscious person at the local baseball field on a very hot (97°F) Saturday. You are accompanied by Steve Phillips, an EMT, your partner for the day, and are en route by 1516.

You arrive on-scene at 1522 to find a young male collapsed at third base. He is unarousable and is perspiring heavily, and his skin is cool to the touch. The pillow under the boy's head (placed by bystanders) is removed, the patient's airway is clear, his breathing is adequate, and his pulse is rapid and bounding. One of the bystanders says the patient was playing ball and just collapsed. Another young bystander identifies himself as the patient's brother and states that "nothing like this has happened before." He says his brother is named Jim Thompson, is 13, and lives about a mile away.

The rest of the assessment reveals no signs of trauma. The assessment findings include blood pressure 136/98; pulse 92 and strong; normal sinus rhythm as revealed by the ECG; respirations 24 and normal in depth and pattern (at 1527). The boy responds to painful stimuli, but not to verbal commands or to his name. Pupils are noted to be equal and slow to react. Oxygen is applied at 12 L per minute by nonrebreather mask, and the patient is moved to the shade.

Receiving Hospital is contacted, and you call in the following report:

_____

_____

_____

_____

_____

_____

_____

_____

_____

_____

Expected ETA at Receiving Hospital is 20 minutes.

Medical direction at Receiving Hospital, the closest facility, orders you to start an IV line with normal saline run just to keep open. You repeat the orders back to medical direction and then begin your care. Your first IV attempt on the right forearm is unsuccessful; the second attempt on the left forearm gets a flashback and infuses well. You retake vitals. The patient is now responding to verbal stimuli, the blood pressure is 134/96, pulse is 90, sinus rhythm is normal via ECG, respirations are 24. The patient is loaded on the stretcher at 1537 and moved to the ambulance.

You contact medical direction and provide the following update:

_____

_____

_____

_____

_____

_____

_____

_____

_____

_____

_____

©2009 Pearson Education, Inc.
Paramedic Care: Principles & Practice, Vol. 2, 3rd. Ed.

ETA is 10 minutes.

En route, vital signs (at 1545) are blood pressure 132/90, normal sinus rhythm via ECG, pulse 88, respirations at 24. The patient is now conscious and alert, though he cannot remember the incident. The trip is uneventful, and you arrive at the hospital at 1557. You transfer the responsibility for the patient to the emergency physician and restock and wipe out the ambulance. You report back into service at 1615, grab a cup of coffee, and sit down at the hospital to write the run report.

Complete the run report on the following page from the information contained in the narrative of this call.

Compare the radio communication and run report form that you prepare against the example in the Answer Key section of this Workbook. As you make the comparison, keep in mind that there are many "correct" ways to communicate this body of information. Be sure that you have recorded the major points of your assessment and care and enough other material to describe the patient and his condition.

Date / /	Emergency Medical Services Run Report	Run # 911

Patient Information	Service Information	Times

Name:	Agency:	Rcvd :
Address:	Location:	Enrt :
City: St: Zip:	Call Origin:	Scne :
Age: Birth: / / Sex: [M][F]	Type: Emrg[ ] Non[ ] Trnsfr[ ]	LvSn :
Nature of Call:		ArHsp :
Chief Complaint:		InSv :

Description of Current Problem:

Medical Problems

Past		Present
[ ]	Cardiac	[ ]
[ ]	Stroke	[ ]
[ ]	Acute Abdomen	[ ]
[ ]	Diabetes	[ ]
[ ]	Psychiatric	[ ]
[ ]	Epilepsy	[ ]
[ ]	Drug/Alcohol	[ ]
[ ]	Poisoning	[ ]
[ ]	Allergy/Asthma	[ ]
[ ]	Syncope	[ ]
[ ]	Obstetrical	[ ]
[ ]	GYN	[ ]

Other:

Trauma Scr: Glasgow:

On-Scene Care:	First Aid:
	By Whom?

0₂ @ L : Via	C-Collar :	S-Immob. :	Stretcher :

Allergies/Meds:	Past Med Hx:

Time	Pulse		Resp.		BP S/D	LOC	ECG
:	R:	[r][i]	R:	[s][l]	/	[a][v][p][u]	
Care/Comments:							
:	R:	[r][i]	R:	[s][l]	/	[a][v][p][u]	
Care/Comments:							
:	R:	[r][i]	R:	[s][l]	/	[a][v][p][u]	
Care/Comments:							
:	R:	[r][i]	R:	[s][l]	/	[a][v][p][u]	
Care/Comments:							

Destination:	Personnel:	Certification
Reason:[ ]pt [ ]Closest [ ]M.D. [ ]Other	1.	[P][E][O]
Contacted: [ ]Radio [ ]Tele [ ]Direct	2.	[P][E][O]
Ar Status: [ ]Better [ ]UnC [ ]Worse	3.	[P][E][O]

©2009 Pearson Education, Inc.
Paramedic Care: Principles & Practice, Vol. 2, 3rd. Ed.

Documentation

Review of Chapter Objectives

After reading this chapter, you should be able to:

1. Identify the general principles regarding the importance of EMS documentation and ways in which documents are used. **pp. 288–290**

The principal EMS document, the prehospital care report (PCR), is the sole permanent written documentation of the response, assessment, care, and transport offered during an emergency call. It is a medical document conveying details of medical care and patient history that remains a part of the patient record, as well as a legal document that may be reviewed in a court of law. The PCR may also be reviewed by medical direction to determine the appropriateness of your actions during the call and used by your service to bill the patient for services. Last, the PCR may be used by researchers to determine the effectiveness of care measures in improving patient outcomes.

2. Identify and properly use medical terminology, medical abbreviations, and acronyms. **pp. 292–297**

Medical terminology is the very precise and exact wording used to describe the human body and injuries or illnesses. Proper use of this terminology turns the PCR into a medical document. However, if terms are misspelled or misused, they may distract from the document and confuse the reader about the patient's condition and the care he has had or should receive. Carry a pocket dictionary, and use words only when you are sure of both their spelling and their usage. The same holds true of medical abbreviations. They must be applied properly and have the same meaning to both the writer and the reader. EMS systems should use a standardized set of abbreviations and acronyms to ensure good and efficient documentation.

3. Explain the role of documentation in agency reimbursement. **p. 289**

Good documentation is essential for ambulance agencies that bill for services they provide. The PCR provides the name and address of the patient, as well as the nature and circumstances of injury and illness. It also includes the care and transport provided. Without this information, the service may not be able to obtain reimbursement for services rendered and, ultimately, to afford to provide the vehicle, equipment, and personnel necessary to provide prehospital emergency care.

4. Identify and eliminate extraneous or nonprofessional information. **p. 302**

The ambulance call should be documented in a brief and professional way. The PCR describing it may be scrutinized by hospital staff, the medical direction physician, quality improvement committees, supervisors, lawyers, and the news media. Any derogatory comments, jargon, slang, biased statements, irrelevant opinions, or libelous statements will distract from the seriousness of the document and from acceptance of the preparer's professionalism.

5. **Describe the differences between subjective and objective elements of documentation.** pp. 302–305

Subjective information is information that you obtain from others or is your opinion that is not based on observable facts. It includes the patient's, family's, or bystander's description of the chief complaint and symptoms, medical history, and nature of the illness or mechanism of injury.

Objective information is information you obtain through direct observation, palpation, auscultation, percussion, or diagnostic evaluation of your patient. It includes the vital signs and the results of the physical exam, including such things as glucose level determination and ECG monitor and pulse oximeter readings.

6. **Evaluate a finished document for errors and omissions proper use and spelling of abbreviations and acronyms.** pp. 299, 301–302

The PCR must contain all information obtainable and necessary for describing the patient's condition recorded in a clearly legible way. The report must be written so that another health care provider can easily understand what is being said and can mentally picture the scene, the patient presentation, the care rendered, and the transport offered by the initial providers. In many cases, what to include in the PCR is a judgment decision made by the care provider, though the report must contain an accurate description of the patient's medical or trauma problem and an accurate and complete history. Correct spelling and use of medical terms is essential and reflects the knowledge of the care provider. Proper use of abbreviations and acronyms can help make the PCR more concise; their improper use, however, may produce ambiguity, confusion, and misunderstanding in readers. Reread the finished PCR and check it carefully before submitting it.

7. **Evaluate the confidential nature of an EMS report.** p. 311

Confidentiality is a patient right, and breaching it can result in severe consequences. Do not discuss or share patient or call information with anyone not involved in the care of the patient. The only exceptions—as necessary—are administration, which may need information for billing; police agencies carrying out criminal investigations; requests for the information under subpoena from a court; and quality assurance committees that may need the information (with the patient's name blocked out) for system review and improvement or for research.

8. **Describe the potential consequences of illegible, incomplete, or inaccurate documentation.** pp. 299, 301–302

A legible, complete, and accurate PCR is essential to call documentation. The information in it must be easy to read thanks to both good penmanship and conscientious attention to detail. The report must describe all the pertinent information gathered at the scene and en route to the hospital, as well as all actions taken by you and others in the care of the patient. Failure to create a thorough, readable PCR reduces the information available to other caregivers and may reduce their ability to provide effective care. The document you produce also reflects on your ability to provide assessment and care and your professionalism in general.

9. **Describe the special documentation considerations concerning patient refusal of care and or transport.** pp. 307–308

Be careful in the documentation of a patient who refuses care or transport. While a conscious and mentally competent patient has the right to refuse care, his doing so may pose legal problems for care providers. Document the nature and severity of the patient's injuries, any care you offered, and any care he refused and document carefully the assessment criteria you used to determine the patient was capable of making the decision to refuse care or transport. Also document the patient's reasons for refusing care and your efforts to convince him to change his mind. If possible, have the refusal of care and your explanation to the patient of the consequences of care refusal signed by the patient and witnessed by family, bystanders, or police. Advise the patient to seek other medical help, such as his family physician, and to call EMS again if he changes his mind or his condition worsens.

©2009 Pearson Education, Inc.
Paramedic Care: Principles & Practice, Vol. 2, 3rd. Ed.

10. **Demonstrate how to properly record direct patient or bystander comments.**   p. 298

Direct statements by patients and bystanders must be recorded exactly as they were made and the key phrases placed in quotation marks. Treating the information this way is highly important because it identifies that the information is directly from the source, not an interpretation. Identify clearly the source of any quotation you include in a PCR.

11. **Describe the special considerations concerning multiple-casualty incident documentation.**   pp. 309–311

Often a multiple casualty situation calls for an atypical EMS response and unusual documentation procedures. Care providers rarely stay with a patient from the beginning to the end of prehospital care, and the time spent at a patient's side is very much at a premium. Therefore, documentation must be efficient and incremental. Document your assessment findings and any interventions you perform at the patient's side quickly and clearly. Many agencies or systems have their own forms, such as triage tags, that simplify the documentation procedure.

12. **Demonstrate proper document revision and correction.**   pp. 301–302

Everyone makes mistakes during a health care career and during the process of care documentation. When this happens, it is essential to make corrections in such a way that there is no appearance of impropriety. If an error is made, draw a single line through the error and enter the correction and your initials. If the error is noted after the report is turned in, write a narrative addendum explaining both the nature of the error and the needed correction and ensure that the addendum is included with all copies of the PCR. Correct errors as soon as possible after they are discovered.

13. **Give a prehospital care report form and a narrative patient care scenario, record all pertinent administrative information using a consistent format; identify and record the pertinent, reportable clinical data for each patient; correct errors and omissions using proper procedures; and note and record "pertinent negative" clinical findings.**   pp. 288–312

During your classroom, clinical, and field training, you will complete various reports, including prehospital care reports, on the real and simulated patients you attend. Use the information presented in this text chapter, the information on documentation presented by your instructors, and the guidance given by your clinical and field preceptors to develop good documentation skills. Continue to refine these skills once your training ends and you begin your career as a paramedic.

Case Study Review

Reread the case study on pages 287 and 288 in Paramedic Care: Patient Assessment *and then read the following discussion.*

This case study identifies some of the important considerations regarding the prehospital care report and its potential to support (or incriminate) a care provider who is called into a court of law. The scenario emphasizes the importance of good documentation as described in Chapter 6.

We seldom realize the importance others may place on our prehospital documentation. In this case study, Tom Brewster is surprised when, 3 years after a call, he is summoned to give a legal deposition about it. While this example speaks to legal reasons for review of documentation, Tom might just as well have been asked about the quickness of the ambulance response, the time he and his crew spent on-scene, or specific aspects of the care he provided. Although attorneys may represent the most feared interrogators to most paramedics, the EMS system medical director, quality improvement personnel, or administrative personnel might also ask for details of an incident months or years in the past. For these reasons, your accurate and thorough documentation of the emergency scene and the assessment and care you provide is of great importance to you and your service.

Tom was asked about his recall of the events of the call and the comments made by the patient. His prehospital care report provided enough information to prompt Tom to remember the incident, the patient, and the care he gave. He was fortunate that his documentation provided this information and that he could piece together the events of that response. It is likely that the patient's attorney would challenge Tom's recall after 3 years. Documentation of the patient's statement that he "fell asleep" would be a factor critical in determining the reason for the crash (ruling out medical causes). Tom was apparently thorough in gathering the patient history and recording it on the PCR, because he was able to recall that there was no history of either diabetes or heart disease. Tom further benefited from performing a routine but complete patient assessment, including glucose testing and ECG monitoring.

This case study emphasizes the importance of preparing a prehospital care report that describes exactly what happened and exactly what you did. Had Tom used sloppy penmanship or subjective statements or failed to provide complete information, the patient's attorney would have been able to challenge Tom's objectivity and accuracy. As things stood, the report supported Tom's recall and evaluation of the patient's condition.

Content Self-Evaluation

MULTIPLE CHOICE

_____ 1. The prehospital care report is likely to be reviewed by which of the following?
   A. researchers
   B. EMS administrators
   C. lawyers
   D. medical professionals
   E. all of the above

_____ 2. Which of the following is NOT an appropriate purpose for reviewing a prehospital care report?
   A. to identify a chronological account of the patient's mental status
   B. to learn about what calls other paramedics had
   C. to help detect patient improvement or deterioration
   D. to identify what bystanders and family said at the scene
   E. to determine baseline assessment findings

_____ 3. The prehospital care report may yield information that the quality improvement committee may use to identify problems with individual paramedics or with the EMS system.
   A. True
   B. False

_____ 4. The prehospital care report should contain all of the following EXCEPT:
   A. a description of your patient's condition when you arrived.
   B. your opinions about the patient's attitude or social/economic situation.
   C. a description of your patient's condition after interventions.
   D. the medical status of your patient upon arrival at the emergency department.
   E. response time to the call.

_____ 5. If you have doubts about the spelling of a term when completing a PCR, use a phonetically close spelling; doing this may still convey the right meaning and will not reflect poorly on your professionalism.
   A. True
   B. False

©2009 Pearson Education, Inc.
Paramedic Care: Principles & Practice, Vol. 2, 3rd. Ed.

_____ 6. Which of the following is NOT a time commonly recorded on the prehospital care report?
   A. call received
   B. dispatch time
   C. arrival at the patient's side
   D. arrival at the scene
   E. departure from the scene

_____ 7. Since your watch, the dispatch clock, and other timing devices are not often synchronized, it is important to record all times on the PCR care report from one clock or watch when possible or to indicate when different clocks are used.
   A. True
   B. False

_____ 8. Which of the following is NOT an example of a pertinent negative?
   A. no shortness of breath in a myocardial infarction patient
   B. no history of epilepsy in a seizing patient
   C. clear breath sounds in a congestive heart failure patient
   D. a blood pressure of 90/60
   E. no jugular vein distention in a congestive heart failure patient

_____ 9. The recommended way of indicating the exact words spoken by a patient or bystander is to:
   A. underline the passage.
   B. draw one line through the center of the word or passage.
   C. begin and end the passage with quotation marks.
   D. place the passage in parentheses.
   E. none of the above.

_____ 10. All of the following describe good documentation EXCEPT:
   A. complete.
   B. altered.
   C. accurate.
   D. objective.
   E. legible.

_____ 11. The PCR is created by the paramedic as a personal record of what happened at the scene and during transport, and thus its legibility to others is not important.
   A. True
   B. False

_____ 12. The benefit of check boxes on a prehospital care report is that they:
   A. ensure that common information is recorded for every call.
   B. eliminate the need for a patient narrative.
   C. address every chief complaint.
   D. speed the completion of the narrative.
   E. all of the above.

_____ 13. When should the prehospital care report be completed?
   A. at the end of the day
   B. at the end of your duty shift
   C. once back at quarters
   D. shortly after leaving the hospital
   E. upon or shortly after transferring patient care at the hospital

_____ 14. Whenever possible, have all members of your crew read or reread the prehospital care report before you submit it.
   A. True
   B. False

_____ 15. What is the best way to add information to the prehospital care report after it has been submitted to the hospital?
   A. Search and make changes on all copies.
   B. Change only the original report.
   C. Create an addendum and add it to all reports.
   D. Never add additional material to the report once distributed.
   E. Send a memorandum to medical direction.

_____ 16. Use of professional jargon in the PCR is an indicator of the writer's professionalism.
   A. True
   B. False

_____ 17. Which of the following is the best example of a subjective and possibly libelous statement?
   A. "The patient smelled of beer."
   B. "The patient walked with a staggering gait."
   C. "The patient used abusive language and spoke with slurred speech."
   D. "The patient was drunk and obnoxious."
   E. None of the above is a potentially libelous statement.

_____ 18. Which of the following is a part of the subjective patient information?
   A. chief complaint
   B. past medical history
   C. history of the current medical problem
   D. patient description of what happened
   E. all of the above

_____ 19. The portion of your narrative report that contains your general impression of the patient is the:
   A. subjective narrative.
   B. objective narrative.
   C. assessment/management plan.
   D. SOAP plan.
   E. none of the above.

_____ 20. You should document a pediatric assessment in head-to-toe order, even though you may have performed it from toe-to-head.
   A. True
   B. False

_____ 21. Which of the following is true about the body systems method of assessment?
   A. It focuses on body systems rather than body areas.
   B. It usually addresses only the system(s) affected.
   C. It is best suited to screening and preadmission exams.
   D. It can be a comprehensive approach to documentation.
   E. All of the above are correct.

_____ 22. The term that describes what you believe to be the patient's most likely problem is:
   A. definitive assessment.
   B. clinical diagnosis.
   C. assessment object.
   D. field diagnosis.
   E. none of the above.

_____ 23. The management portion of your documentation should include which of the following?
   A. any interventions
   B. the results of ongoing assessments
   C. any changes in the patient's condition
   D. the patient's condition when care is transferred at the emergency department
   E. all of the above

©2009 Pearson Education, Inc.
Paramedic Care: Principles & Practice, Vol. 2, 3rd. Ed.

_____ 24. Which of the following is NOT a part of the subjective information recorded on the PCR?
   A. vital signs
   B. past medical history
   C. review of systems
   D. chief complaint
   E. none of the above

_____ 25. Which of the following is an element of the objective information recorded on the PCR?
   A. your general impression of the patient
   B. the results of any diagnostic tests
   C. the results of the physical exam
   D. vital signs
   E. all of the above

_____ 26. Which of the following formats records the chief complaint, history, assessment, treatment, and transport information, in that order?
   A. SOAP format
   B. CHART format
   C. patient management format
   D. call incident format
   E. none of the above

_____ 27. The most significant feature of the patient management format of documentation is that it
   A. documents the chronological sequence of events and actions.
   B. focuses exclusively on assessment findings.
   C. uses a free-flowing narrative style.
   D. is most frequently used for patients with minor injuries/problems.
   E. none of the above.

_____ 28. The call incident format for documenting an emergency response is best suited for which type of patient?
   A. the unresponsive medical patient
   B. the responsive medical patient
   C. the trauma patient with no significant mechanism of injury
   D. the trauma patient with a significant mechanism of injury
   E. both B and C

_____ 29. In obtaining a patient refusal against medical advice, it is important to:
   A. determine that the patient is alert, oriented, and competent to make the decision.
   B. clearly explain to the patient the risks of not receiving care.
   C. try to convince the patient to obtain care.
   D. explain that, if the condition worsens, the patient should call for the ambulance or otherwise seek immediate care.
   E. all of the above.

_____ 30. If your ambulance call is canceled en route to the scene, you should:
   A. simply return to base.
   B. write "canceled" on the front of the PCR.
   C. note the canceling authority and time of cancellation on the PCR.
   D. secure the name of the patient as well as any other information.
   E. none of the above.

MATCHING

Write the letter of the word or phrase in the space provided next to the appropriate abbreviation.

_____ 31. CC		A.	shortness of breath
_____ 32. y/o		B.	acute myocardial infarction
_____ 33. wt		C.	positive end-expiratory pressure
_____ 34. CNS		D.	normal sinus rhythm
_____ 35. SOB		E.	nausea/vomiting
_____ 36. n/v		F.	Do Not Resuscitate
_____ 37. AMI		G.	breath sounds/blood sugar
_____ 38. CHF		H.	premature ventricular contraction
_____ 39. ICP		I.	not applicable
_____ 40. MVC		J.	nitroglycerin
_____ 41. STD		K.	intraosseous
_____ 42. NTG		L.	weight
_____ 43. LLQ		M.	sexually transmitted disease
_____ 44. BS		N.	against medical advice
_____ 45. ECG		O.	congestive heart failure
_____ 46. JVD		P.	chief complaint
_____ 47. n/a		Q.	left lower quadrant
_____ 48. AMA		R.	electrocardiogram
_____ 49. DNR		S.	to keep open
_____ 50. PEEP		T.	central nervous system
_____ 51. Tx		U.	intracranial pressure
_____ 52. IO		V.	jugular vein distention
_____ 53. TKO		W.	treatment
_____ 54. NSR		X.	motor vehicle crash
_____ 55. PVC		Y.	year old

Special Project

Documentation: Radio Report/Prehospital Care Report

The preparation of both the radio message to medical direction and writing of the written run report are two of the most important tasks you will perform as a paramedic. Read the following information, compose your initial and updated radio messages, and then complete the run report for this call.

The Call

At 1832, medic rescue Unit 21 is paged through dispatch and is en route to a one-car collision at the corner of Elm and Wildwood Lanes. One patient is reported unconscious, and

©2009 Pearson Education, Inc.
Paramedic Care: Principles & Practice, Vol. 2, 3rd. Ed.

the fire department is also en route. You and your partner, Mike Grailing (a paramedic), arrive with the ambulance at 1845 and find that there are wires down, fuel spilling from the gas tank, and window glass around the scene. Bystanders state that the car swerved wildly, then hit the power pole. You notice there are no skid marks. You stand by, awaiting arrival of the fire department and the securing of the scene.

Once the scene is safe, your partner employs a jaw-thrust with cervical precautions and applies cervical stabilization, while you apply the cervical collar (1850) and begin the assessment. You notice a break in the car's windshield and a small contusion on your patient's forehead. He is unconscious, has a strong pulse, and displays some respiratory wheezing and stridor. Assessment of the neck reveals a small welt but no other apparent injuries. The pupils are equal and reactive. Oxygen is administered at 12 L per minute via nonrebreather mask, the patient awakens, and initial vitals (including a respiratory rate of 30 with audible wheezes, blood pressure of 110/76, a strong pulse of 90, and oxygen saturation of 94 percent) are taken at 1852. The ECG displays normal sinus rhythm.

The patient awakens and asks, "What happened?" He states that he thinks he was stung by a bee. Two years ago he had a similar sting and reaction and has a kit at home that his physician prescribed for him. He is experiencing itching, and there are noticeable hives. He says he feels like "I have a lump in my throat."

Based upon protocol, you initiate the IV run TKO with lactated Ringer's solution in the right forearm using a 16-gauge over-the-catheter needle while the patient is being immobilized and moved to a long spine board.

Medical direction is contacted and you call in the following:

_____

_____

_____

_____

_____

_____

_____

_____

_____

_____

_____

_____

_____

Orders for 0.3 mg epinephrine subcutaneously (1:1,000) and 50 mg Benadryl IM are received, and the medications are administered at 1855. Just prior to moving the patient to the ambulance, the patient is monitored and found to have the following vitals: blood pressure 118/88, pulse 78 strong and regular, respirations 20 and regular with clear breath sounds, an ECG showing normal sinus rhythm, and a pulse oximetry reading of 99 percent.

The patient history, which is taken at the scene and during transport, reveals that the patient's name is William Sobeski, his age is 28, and he lives at 2145 East Brookline Drive in the city of Rochester. The patient denies any allergy, except to bee stings. He was stung by a bee 2 years ago and was rushed to the emergency department because he "couldn't catch his breath." He denies any headache, visual disturbances, and numbness and tingling.

He also denies taking any prescribed medications and has not eaten since noon. The patient requests Community Hospital because his sister works there. En route, vitals are blood pressure 122/78, pulse of 68 strong and regular, respirations 22 and regular, and a pulse oximetry reading of 98 percent, all taken at 1902.

Contact medical direction and provide the following update:

_____

_____

_____

_____

_____

_____

_____

_____

ETA is 10 minutes.

The final vitals, taken just before arrival, are blood pressure 122/80, pulse 86, oxygen saturation of 98 percent, and respirations 24 and regular with no wheezes. The ECG still displays normal sinus rhythm, and the patient is conscious and oriented. He states that the feeling of a lump in the throat is gone.

The trip is uneventful, and the patient is delivered to the emergency department at 1925. The patient care responsibilities are transferred to the staff, and the attending physician is given the final patient update. The vehicle is restocked and cleaned, and you are ready for service at 1955.

Using the information contained in this narrative, complete the run report on the next page.

Compare the radio communication and run report form that you prepared against the example in the Answer Key section of this Workbook. As you make this comparison, keep in mind that there are many "correct" ways to communicate this body of information. Ensure that the information you have recorded contains the major points of your assessment and care and enough other material to describe the patient and his condition to the receiving physician and anyone else who might review the form. Remember that this document may be the only record of your assessment and care for this patient. When you are done, it should be a complete account of your actions.

©2009 Pearson Education, Inc.
Paramedic Care: Principles & Practice, Vol. 2, 3rd. Ed.

| Date / / | Emergency Medical Services Run Report | Run # 911 |

Patient Information

| Name: |
| Address: |
| City: | St: | Zip: |
| Age: | Birth: / / | Sex: [M][F] |
| Nature of Call: |
| Chief Complaint: |

Service Information

| Agency: |
| Location: |
| Call Origin: |
| Type: Emrg[ ] Non[ ] Trnsfr[ ] |

Times

Rcvd	:
Enrt	:
Scne	:
LvSn	:
ArHsp	:
InSv	:

Description of Current Problem:

Medical Problems

Past		Present
[ ]	Cardiac	[ ]
[ ]	Stroke	[ ]
[ ]	Acute Abdomen	[ ]
[ ]	Diabetes	[ ]
[ ]	Psychiatric	[ ]
[ ]	Epilepsy	[ ]
[ ]	Drug/Alcohol	[ ]
[ ]	Poisoning	[ ]
[ ]	Allergy/Asthma	[ ]
[ ]	Syncope	[ ]
[ ]	Obstetrical	[ ]
[ ]	GYN	[ ]

Other:

Trauma Scr: Glasgow:

On-Scene Care:	First Aid:
	By Whom?

| 0₂ @   L   :   Via | C-Collar   : | S-Immob.   : | Stretcher   : |

| Allergies/Meds: | Past Med Hx: |

Time	Pulse	Resp.	BP S/D	LOC	ECG
:	R: [r][i]	R: [s][l]	/	[a][v][p][u]	
Care/Comments:					
:	R: [r][i]	R: [s][l]	/	[a][v][p][u]	
Care/Comments:					
:	R: [r][i]	R: [s][l]	/	[a][v][p][u]	
Care/Comments:					
:	R: [r][i]	R: [s][l]	/	[a][v][p][u]	
Care/Comments:					

Destination:	Personnel:	Certification
Reason:[ ]pt [ ]Closest [ ]M.D. [ ]Other	1.	[P][E][O]
Contacted: [ ]Radio [ ]Tele [ ]Direct	2.	[P][E][O]
Ar Status: [ ]Better [ ]UnC [ ]Worse	3.	[P][E][O]

PATIENT ASSESSMENT
Content Review
Content Self-Evaluation

Chapter I: The History

____ 1. The listing of possible causes of your patient's symptoms or chief complaint is the:
   A. presenting problem.
   B. field diagnosis.
   C. differential field diagnosis.
   D. chief complaint.
   E. summary diagnosis.

____ 2. Making a proper first impression involves:
   A. developing trust between the care provider and patient.
   B. developing a positive patient/care provider relationship.
   C. establishing the professionalism of the care provider.
   D. calming and reassuring the patient.
   E. all of the above.

____ 3. Which of the following is NOT a recommended action during your introduction to the patient?
   A. assuming a position at the patient's eye level
   B. addressing your patient by a familiar name, such as "Pops" or "Dear"
   C. dressing in a fresh, clean uniform
   D. introducing yourself by name, title, and agency
   E. using your patient's name frequently

____ 4. Which of the following is an example of an open-ended question?
   A. Does your pain increase with breathing?
   B. Have you experienced this problem before?
   C. Do you take any medications for your condition?
   D. Does the pain radiate to your shoulder?
   E. Where do you hurt?

____ 5. Which of the following questions is an example of a closed-ended question?
   A. Has this happened to you before?
   B. How would you describe your pain?
   C. What were you doing when this problem began?
   D. What medications are you on?
   E. All of the above are correct.

____ 6. The interviewing technique in which you restate the patient's words is:
   A. reflection.
   B. clarification.
   C. active listening.
   D. confrontation.
   E. interpretation.

_____ 7. The interviewing technique represented by the statement to the patient "You say you feel fine, but you seem uneasy and uncomfortable" is:
A. distraction.
B. reflection.
C. facilitation.
D. confrontation.
E. clarification.

_____ 8. The pain, discomfort, or dysfunction that causes the patient to summon emergency medical service is the:
A. primary problem.
B. chief complaint.
C. nature of the illness.
D. mechanism of injury.
E. none of the above.

_____ 9. The absence of dyspnea in a patient experiencing chest pain would be an example of which of the OPQRST-ASPN components of the history of the current illness?
A. O
B. P
C. T
D. AS
E. PN

_____ 10. The CAGE questionnaire is used in questioning a patient about:
A. alcoholism.
B. chest pain.
C. dyspnea.
D. "caine" family allergies.
E. current medication use.

_____ 11. Which of the following represents a 10 pack/year smoker?
A. 1 pack per day for 5 years
B. 2 packs per day for 5 years
C. 4 packs per day for 5 years
D. 1 pack per day for 10 years
E. both B and D

_____ 12. Which of the following previous family conditions is not important in determining the family history?
A. asthma
B. cardiac problems
C. traumatic death
D. allergies
E. hypertension

_____ 13. The term "para" refers to which of the following regarding the obstetrical status of a female patient?
A. number of pregnancies
B. number of viable births
C. number of abortions
D. number of living children
E. none of the above

_____ 14. The first priority in caring for a belligerent and intoxicated patient is:
A. having friends and family present.
B. creating a calming environment.
C. having enough personnel present to restrain the patient.
D. ensuring a safe environment.
E. using appropriate clinical judgment.

_____ 15. Most patients comment on and remember the technical skills and abilities of the paramedics who treat them.
A. True
B. False

©2009 Pearson Education, Inc.
Paramedic Care: Principles & Practice, Vol. 2, 3rd. Ed.

Chapter 2: Physical Exam Techniques

____ 16. Hyperresonance would be discovered during assessment using the technique of:
A. palpation.
B. auscultation.
C. inspection.
D. percussion.
E. none of the above.

____ 17. To evaluate a patient's skin temperature, it is best to use the:
A. tips of the fingers.
B. pads of the fingers.
C. palm of the hands.
D. back of the hands or fingers.
E. none of the above.

____ 18. To evaluate tissue masses, it is best to use the:
A. tips of the fingers.
B. pads of the fingers.
C. palm of the hands.
D. back of the hands or fingers.
E. none of the above.

____ 19. To employ deep palpation, apply pressure and sense using the fingers of only one hand, which will increase your sensitivity to masses, guarding, and other pathologies.
A. True
B. False

____ 20. The thudding sound produced by percussing a solid organ, such as the liver, is described as:
A. hyperresonance.   D. flat.
B. dull.   E. none of the above.
C. resonance.

____ 21. Tachycardia is likely to be caused by all of the following EXCEPT:
A. fever.   D. hypoxia.
B. pain.   E. sympathetic stimulation.
C. hypothermia.

____ 22. The process of normal inspiration is:
A. an active action involving accessory muscles.
B. an active action involving the diaphragm and intercostal muscles.
C. active in its early stages and passive in its later stages.
D. passive in its early stages and active in its later stages.
E. passive.

____ 23. The pressure of the blood within the blood vessels caused by contraction of the ventricles is the:
A. Korotkoff pressure.
B. systolic pressure.
C. diastolic pressure.
D. asystolic pressure.
E. atrial pressure.

____ 24. The pulse pressure of a patient with a pulse rate of 72, a blood pressure of 120/90, and a respiratory rate of 16 is:
A. 18.   D. 90.
B. 30.   E. 120.
C. 72.

_____ 25. The average blood pressure in a healthy adult is:
A. 90/60.   D. 140/90.
B. 100/70.   E. 180/100.
C. 120/80.

_____ 26. The normal respiratory tidal volume for a healthy adult is about:
A. 100 mL.   D. 800 mL.
B. 200 mL.   E. 1,200 mL.
C. 500 mL.

_____ 27. The systolic blood pressure represents a measure of:
A. peripheral vascular resistance.
B. the cardiac output.
C. the viscosity of the blood.
D. the strength of ventricular contraction.
E. relative blood volume.

_____ 28. Hypotension is defined as:
A. a systolic blood pressure below 100.
B. a diastolic blood pressure below 60.
C. a blood pressure below 100/60.
D. either a diastolic pressure below 70 or a systolic pressure below 90.
E. a lower than normal blood pressure.

_____ 29. To facilitate the conduction of high-pitched sounds through the stethoscope bell, apply the bell using:
A. firm pressure.
B. moderate pressure.
C. light pressure.
D. alternating firm and light pressure.
E. no pressure at all.

_____ 30. In a patient with a weak and irregular pulse, determine the pulse rate by assessing the number of beats in:
A. 2 minutes and dividing by 2.
B. 1 minute.
C. 30 seconds and multiplying by 2.
D. 15 seconds and multiplying by 4.
E. 10 seconds and multiplying by 5.

_____ 31. The width of a correctly sized sphygmomanometer cuff should be:
A. one-half to one-third the circumference of the patient's arm.
B. one-half to one-third the radius of the patient's arm.
C. two-thirds the length of the patient's upper arm.
D. one-third the length of the patient's upper arm.
E. either A or C.

_____ 32. When taking blood pressure, deflate the cuff at a rate of:
A. 2 to 3 mmHg per heartbeat.
B. 4 to 6 mmHg per heartbeat.
C. 5 to 10 mmHg per heartbeat.
D. 8 to 12 mmHg per heartbeat.
E. 10 to 20 mmHg per heartbeat.

_____ 33. As the blood pressure cuff is deflated, the first pulse beat heard through the stethoscope represents the:
A. Kussmaul sound.   D. pulse pressure.
B. diastolic blood pressure.   E. Doppler sound.
C. systolic blood pressure.

©2009 Pearson Education, Inc.
Paramedic Care: Principles & Practice, Vol. 2, 3rd. Ed.

____ 34. The pulse oximeter reading indicates:
   A. carbon dioxide levels in the blood.
   B. inspired air oxygen levels.
   C. expired air oxygen levels.
   D. blood levels of desaturated hemoglobin.
   E. arterial blood oxygen saturation levels.

____ 35. Cyanosis is caused by an increase in:
   A. blood oxygen.
   B. deoxyhemoglobin.
   C. dissolved carbon dioxide.
   D. carboxyhemoglobin.
   E. natural coloration overshadowing the red of blood.

____ 36. The discoloration that represents a blue hue is:
   A. cyanosis.
   B. jaundice.
   C. sckophosis.
   D. erythema.
   E. carotanemia.

____ 37. A heavy and greasy scaling of the skin under the hair is:
   A. dandruff.
   B. nits.
   C. seborrheic dermatitis.
   D. psoriasis.
   E. none of the above.

____ 38. The bluish discoloration just around the eyes is suggestive of a basilar skull fracture.
   A. True
   B. False

____ 39. The dark opening in the center of the eye that constricts and dilates to regulate the amount of light falling on the optic surface is the:
   A. retina.
   B. pupil.
   C. conjunctiva.
   D. sclera.
   E. lens.

____ 40. The term that describes fine jerking movements of the eye is:
   A. hypopyon.
   B. hyphema.
   C. conjunctival hemorrhage.
   D. anisocoria.
   E. nystagmus.

____ 41. The term for the common runny nose is:
   A. epistaxis.
   B. otorrhea.
   C. rhinorrhea.
   D. rhinitis.
   E. none of the above.

____ 42. The layer of tissue that covers the exterior of the lung and helps ensure that the lungs move with the thorax is the:
   A. visceral pleura.
   B. parietal pleura.
   C. peritoneum.
   D. pulmonary pleura.
   E. perineum.

____ 43. A location where you are NOT likely to notice retractions during forced inspiration is the:
   A. suprasternal notch.
   B. intercostal spaces.
   C. supraclavicular space.
   D. costal border.
   E. both A and C.

____ 44. A finding of decreased tactile fremitus suggests:
   A. pneumonia.
   B. a tumor.
   C. pulmonary fibrosis.
   D. emphysema.
   E. none of the above.

_____ 45. Which condition is most likely to cause an area of the lung that is hyperresonant to percussion?
A. pneumothorax
B. pneumonia
C. hemothorax
D. pericardial tamponade
E. friction rubs

_____ 46. The high-pitched, continuous, almost musical notes heard during chest auscultation of the asthma patient are:
A. rhonchi.
B. stridor.
C. crackles.
D. wheezes.
E. none of the above.

_____ 47. The "dub" of the heart sounds represents which event of the cardiac cycle?
A. ejection of blood from the ventricles
B. ventricular contraction
C. ventricular filling
D. closing of the aortic and pulmonic valves
E. closing of the tricuspid and mitral valves

_____ 48. The sound of turbulent blood flow through an artery is a:
A. trill.
B. murmur.
C. friction rub.
D. bruit.
E. gallop.

_____ 49. Which of the following abdominal organs is located, at least partially, in the right upper quadrant?
A. gallbladder
B. transverse colon
C. pancreas
D. ascending colon
E. all of the above

_____ 50. An ecchymotic discoloration over the flanks is:
A. Grey-Turner's sign.
B. borborygmi.
C. Hering-Breuer sign.
D. Cullen's sign.
E. none of the above.

_____ 51. Assessment of the musculoskeletal system involves:
A. examination of the passive range of motion.
B. examination of the range of motion against gravity.
C. examination of the range of motion against resistance.
D. inspection and palpation.
E. all of the above.

_____ 52. The movement permitted between the metacarpals and phalanges is:
A. abduction/adduction.
B. rotation.
C. flexion/extension.
D. supination/pronation.
E. both A and C.

_____ 53. To test for carpal tunnel syndrome, acutely flex the wrist for 1 minute and expect to have the patient complain of:
A. sharp pain.
B. numbness and tingling.
C. a burning sensation.
D. dull pain.
E. crampy pain referred to axilla.

_____ 54. The most frequently dislocated joint in the human body is the:
A. shoulder.
B. wrist.
C. hip.
D. elbow.
E. ankle.

©2009 Pearson Education, Inc.
Paramedic Care: Principles & Practice, Vol. 2, 3rd. Ed.

_____ 55. The most common sprains of the ankle are:
   A. medial.
   B. lateral.
   C. rotational.
   D. flexional.
   E. extensional.

_____ 56. Which types of motion are permitted by the cervical spine?
   A. rotation
   B. lateral bending
   C. flexion
   D. extension
   E. all of the above

_____ 57. The bony projection of the axis (C2) that the atlas (C1) pivots around is the:
   A. trochar.
   B. ischial tuberosity.
   C. olecranon process.
   D. odontoid process.
   E. none of the above.

_____ 58. An exaggerated curvature of the lumbar spine is:
   A. lordosis.
   B. scoliosis.
   C. kyphosis.
   D. spina bifida.
   E. none of the above.

_____ 59. A bounding pulse quality would be reported as:
   A. 0.
   B. 1+.
   D. 3+.
   E. 4+.

_____ 60. Which of the following is NOT a sign of proximal arterial occlusion?
   A. cold limb
   B. pulse deficit
   C. irregular pulse
   D. poor color in the fingertips
   E. slow capillary refill

_____ 61. The cerebral cortex is the center for which of the following?
   A. rational thought
   B. behavior
   C. speech
   D. language
   E. all of the above

_____ 62. Pitting edema that depresses 1/4 to 1/2 inch is reported as:
   A. 0.
   B. 1+.
   C. 2+.
   D. 3+.
   E. 4+.

_____ 63. The term "dysarthria" refers to:
   A. defective speech caused by motor deficits.
   B. voice changes due to vocal cord problems.
   C. defective language due to neurologic problems.
   D. voice changes due to aging.
   E. joint pain and stiffness.

_____ 64. A patient who responds to stimulation only for short periods is:
   A. lethargic.
   B. obtunded.
   C. stuporous.
   D. comatose.
   E. none of the above.

_____ 65. A question about what a patient had for lunch tests which of the following types of memory?
   A. immediate
   B. verifiable
   C. recent
   D. remote
   E. none of the above

____ 66. The cranial nerve that controls pupillary constriction is which of the following?
   A. CN-I
   B. CN-II
   C. CN-III
   D. CN-VII
   E. CN-X

____ 67. There are how many cranial nerves?
   A. 4 pairs
   B. 6 pairs
   C. 10 pairs
   D. 12 pairs
   E. 16 pairs

____ 68. The cranial nerve responsible for the sense of smell is which of the following?
   A. CN-I
   B. CN-II
   C. CN-III
   D. CN-VII
   E. CN-X

____ 69. The cranial nerve that controls most facial muscles is which of the following?
   A. CN-I
   B. CN-II
   C. CN-III
   D. CN-VII
   E. CN-X

____ 70. When a person loses the sense of balance, which cranial nerve has probably been injured?
   A. equilibrial
   B. glossopharyngeal
   C. acoustic
   D. vagus
   E. accessory

____ 71. When your patient loses balance while standing with eyes closed, that finding is referred to as a(n):
   A. positive Romberg test.
   B. expressive aphasia.
   C. sensory aphasia.
   D. negative Romberg test.
   E. vertigo.

____ 72. To perform the "tandem walking" test, have a patient:
   A. walk heel-to-toe in a straight line.
   B. stand with eyes closed for 20 to 30 seconds.
   C. walk across the room, turn, and walk back again.
   D. do a shallow knee bend on each leg in turn.
   E. walk first on his heels, then toes.

____ 73. To assess the sensory system, you must test for:
   A. pain.
   B. light touch.
   C. temperature.
   D. vibration.
   E. all of the above.

____ 74. Which of the following is NOT recommended as part of the assessment and care for an ill or injured child?
   A. Separate the patient from the parents, if possible.
   B. Give the patient a toy or another object to play with.
   C. Elicit a parent's help in obtaining a history.
   D. Perform invasive procedures late in the assessment, if possible.
   E. Provide feedback and reassurance.

____ 75. In what age group do children usually learn to walk?
   A. infant
   B. toddler
   C. preschooler
   D. school age
   E. adolescent

©2009 Pearson Education, Inc.
Paramedic Care: Principles & Practice, Vol. 2, 3rd. Ed.

____ 76. Which group of children is most worried about mutilation and disfigurement?
A. infant
B. toddler
C. preschooler
D. school age
E. adolescent

____ 77. Bulging along the sutures of the young child's skull suggests which of the following?
A. meningitis
B. head injury
C. increasing intracranial pressure
D. all of the above
E. none of the above

____ 78. Because the chest muscles are underdeveloped, young children are diaphragmatic breathers.
A. True
B. False

____ 79. The normal systolic blood pressure for a preschooler is:
A. 60 to 90 mmHg.
B. 87 to 105 mmHg.
C. 95 to 105 mmHg.
D. 95 to 110 mmHg.
E. 112 to 128 mmHg.

____ 80. The normal pulse rate for an infant is:
A. 60 to 90 per minute.
B. 65 to 110 per minute.
C. 80 to 110 per minute.
D. 100 to 160 per minute.
E. 100 to 180 per minute.

____ 81. The normal respiratory rate for a toddler is:
A. 30 to 50 per minute.
B. 30 to 60 per minute.
C. 24 to 40 per minute.
D. 22 to 34 per minute.
E. 18 to 30 per minute.

____ 82. Which of the following is NOT true regarding the abdomen of the child?
A. The liver is proportionally larger than that of the adult.
B. The spleen is well hidden beneath the rib cage.
C. The abdominal muscles afford less protection than those of the adult.
D. The abdomen bulges at the end of inspiration.
E. Inguinal hernias are common in young male children.

____ 83. The patient's current health status is recorded under which element of the SOAP documentation format?
A. S
B. O
C. A
D. P
E. none of the above

____ 84. The results of auscultation are recorded under which element of the SOAP documentation format?
A. S
B. O
C. A
D. P
E. none of the above

Chapter 3: Patient Assessment in the Field

____ 85. As a paramedic, you will frequently perform a comprehensive physical exam in the acute setting:
A. True
B. False

____ 86. The component of the patient assessment process in which immediate life threats should be identified and corrected is the:
A. scene size-up.
B. initial assessment.
C. focused history and physical exam.
D. detailed physical exam.
E. ongoing assessment.

____ 87. Which of the following is NOT a component of the scene size-up?
A. taking standard precautions
B. locating all patients
C. analyzing the mechanism of injury/nature of the illness
D. determining the priority for transport
E. identifying scene hazards

____ 88. The personal protective equipment you should wear when planning to intubate a patient includes:
A. latex or vinyl gloves and a gown.
B. protective eyewear, a gown, and a face mask.
C. protective eyewear and a gown.
D. latex or vinyl gloves, protective eyewear, and a face mask.
E. latex or vinyl gloves.

____ 89. All of the following circumstances noted during scene size-up should lead you to expect more than one patient EXCEPT:
A. carbon monoxide poisoning in an apartment building.
B. a child seat and diaper bag in a car crash.
C. injury incurred during a tackle in a football game.
D. twin spider webs in the windshield of a crashed car.
E. a hazardous spill in a high school chemistry lab.

____ 90. Two important functions that must begin immediately in the mass casualty situation are:
A. rescue and triage.
B. firefighting and rescue.
C. triage and incident management.
D. incident management and extrication.
E. incident management and scene isolation.

____ 91. The initial assessment includes all of the following steps EXCEPT:
A. forming a general patient impression.
B. gathering a focused patient history.
C. assessing breathing.
D. assessing airway.
E. assessing circulation.

____ 92. The general patient impression is based upon all of the following EXCEPT:
A. patient gender and age.
B. mechanism of injury.
C. chief complaint.
D. oxygen saturation.
E. your instincts.

©2009 Pearson Education, Inc.
Paramedic Care: Principles & Practice, Vol. 2, 3rd. Ed.

___ 93. During the initial assessment, you should stabilize the cervical spine:
   A. immediately, if suggested by the MOI.
   B. after the airway is established.
   C. just before you attempt artificial ventilation.
   D. after the circulation check.
   E. as the last step of the primary survey.

___ 94. A patient who does not respond to a painful stimulus is classified as which of the following under the AVPU system?
   A. A
   B. V
   C. P
   D. U
   E. cannot be determined with the information at hand

___ 95. A patient who awakens to a loud shout is classified as which of the following under the AVPU system?
   A. A
   B. V
   C. P
   D. U
   E. cannot be determined with the information at hand

___ 96. If your patient is responsive and can speak clearly, you can assume that his airway is patent.
   A. True
   B. False

___ 97. The presence of a carotid pulse suggests that the systolic blood pressure is at least:
   A. 60 mmHg.   D. 100 mmHg.
   B. 70 mmHg.   E. 120 mmHg.
   C. 80 mmHg.

___ 98. The focused history and physical exam is conducted differently for the four major categories of patients. Which of the following is NOT one of those categories?
   A. trauma patient with an isolated injury
   B. trauma patient with altered LOC/significant MOI
   C. pediatric patient with altered consciousness
   D. responsive medical patient
   E. unresponsive medical patient

___ 99. Which of the following is NOT a mechanism of injury that calls for rapid transport to the trauma center?
   A. fall from a height greater than 20 feet
   B. moderate vehicle deformity
   C. death of another vehicle occupant
   D. penetration of trunk or head
   E. motorcycle crash

___ 100. If you arrive at your patient's side only moments after the accident, he may not have bled enough to demonstrate the signs of progressive head injury.
   A. True
   B. False

___ 101. Assume your patient has a spinal injury if you find:
   A. a significant mechanism of injury.
   B. an injury above the shoulders.
   C. complaints of numbness.
   D. pain along the spinal column.
   E. all of the above.

102. The "C" of DCAP-BTLS stands for:
    A. cuts.
    B. cutaneous injury.
    C. circulatory deficit.
    D. contusions.
    E. carotid bruits.

103. Fracture and manipulation of the clavicle are likely to lead to:
    A. subclavian artery injury.
    B. subclavian vein injury.
    C. hemothorax.
    D. pneumothorax.
    E. all of the above.

104. During the rapid trauma assessment, it is important to evaluate the abdomen carefully to determine the exact nature of the injury and then take the necessary care steps.
    A. True
    B. False

105. The "P" of the SAMPLE history stands for:
    A. past medical history.
    B. palpated deformities.
    C. precipitating factors.
    D. pulse deficits.
    E. pupillary responses.

106. The field diagnosis for a medical patient is most frequently determined from:
    A. the physical assessment.
    B. the patient's story.
    C. the SAMPLE history.
    D. the vital signs.
    E. none of the above.

107. Which of the following is a part of the patient history?
    A. chief complaint
    B. history of the present illness
    C. past medical history
    D. current health status
    E. all of the above

108. A patient statement that "he has substernal and left arm pain" would fall under what element of the OPQRST-ASPN mnemonic for investigation of the chief complaint?
    A. O   D. S
    B. P   E. PN
    C. R

109. Which of the following is NOT likely to cause jugular vein distention?
    A. cardiac tamponade
    B. tension pneumothorax
    C. right heart failure
    D. hemothorax
    E. All of the above may cause distention.

110. If you hear diffuse expiratory wheezing while auscultating a patient's chest, you should suspect:
    A. congestive heart failure.
    B. pulmonary edema.
    C. asthma.
    D. pulmonary embolism.
    E. all of the above.

©2009 Pearson Education, Inc.
Paramedic Care: Principles & Practice, Vol. 2, 3rd. Ed.

____ 111. The ECG allows you to determine all of the following EXCEPT:
  A. cardiac rate.
  B. cardiac rhythm.
  C. cardiac output.
  D. sequencing of the cardiac events.
  E. All of the above can be determined by the ECG.

____ 112. Which of the following patients is likely to receive the most comprehensive assessment?
  A. trauma patient with a significant mechanism of injury
  B. trauma patient with an isolated injury
  C. unresponsive medical patient
  D. responsive medical patient
  E. any unconscious patient

____ 113. You would normally expect to perform the detailed physical assessment on the serious trauma or medical patient:
  A. early in on-scene assessment and care.
  B. en route to the hospital.
  C. late in on-scene assessment and care.
  D. on-scene for medical patients only.
  E. never.

Chapter 4: Clinical Decision Making

____ 114. The paramedics of the twenty-first century will be highly trained and practiced field technicians working under rigid protocols.
  A. True
  B. False

____ 115. Which of the following is NOT a level of patient acuity?
  A. a critically life-threatening condition
  B. a nonlife-threatening condition
  C. a potentially nonlife-threatening condition
  D. a potentially life-threatening condition
  E. none of the above

____ 116. A standard of emergency care approved by the system medical director is a(n):
  A. protocol.
  B. standing order.
  C. algorithm.
  D. special care enhancement.
  E. none of the above.

____ 117. To employ critical decision-making skills as a paramedic, you must first have an:
  A. excellent working knowledge of pathophysiology.
  B. excellent working knowledge of anatomy and physiology.
  C. understanding of the role each body system plays in overall body function.
  D. ability to analyze numerous signs and symptoms associated with the disease.
  E. all of the above.

____ 118. The key to remaining calm and functioning well under the stress of an emergency is to
  A. focus on the task and block out distractions.
  B. let others know you are struggling and need help.
  C. stay away from a systematic approach because emergencies are usually unanticipated.
  D. employ one management style and stick with it.
  E. all of the above.

____ 119. The thinking style in which all aspects of a situation are considered before arriving at a solution is:
   A. reflective.
   B. impulsive.
   C. divergent.
   D. convergent.
   E. anticipatory.

____ 120. The body system that may interfere with your ability to think critically at the emergency scene is the:
   A. cardiovascular system.
   B. respiratory system.
   C. somatic nervous system.
   D. autonomic nervous system.
   E. renal system.

____ 121. The portion of the mental checklist approach to emergency care in which you consider all options before employing an emergency care modality is:
   A. scan the situation.
   B. stop and think.
   C. decide and act.
   D. maintain control.
   E. reevaluate.

Chapter 5: Communications

____ 122. The basic communications model of exchange of information includes which of the following?
   A. sender encoding a message
   B. sender transmitting a message
   C. receiver decoding a message
   D. receiver providing feedback
   E. all of the above

____ 123. The radio band that penetrates buildings and is less susceptible to interference is:
   A. VHF low-band.
   B. VHF high-band.
   C. UHF.
   D. microwave.
   E. none of the above.

____ 124. The prehospital care report should NOT be used by:
   A. administration for billing.
   B. the emergency department staff to identify your patient findings.
   C. quality assurance committees to improve system function.
   D. other paramedics to identify your interesting calls.
   E. the insurance department for billing.

____ 125. The phase of the emergency communications system that uses the telephone most heavily is:
   A. detection and citizen access.
   B. the emergency response.
   C. call coordination and incident recording.
   D. discussion with medical direction.
   E. transfer communications.

©2009 Pearson Education, Inc.
Paramedic Care: Principles & Practice, Vol. 2, 3rd. Ed.

_____ 126. The system that uses caller questioning and established guidelines to determine the types of units that respond to a particular emergency is:
A. system status management.
B. priority dispatching.
C. code identification.
D. EMD.
E. none of the above.

_____ 127. The radio transmission design that does not permit the receiver to interrupt the caller while he is talking is:
A. simplex.
B. duplex.
C. multiplex.
D. trunking.
E. none of the above.

_____ 128. Which of the following is NOT true regarding digital communication?
A. It is clearer than analog.
B. It is faster than analog.
C. It may increase overcrowding of radio frequencies.
D. It cannot be monitored by a standard scanner.
E. It is becoming increasingly popular for EMS communications.

_____ 129. All of the following are appropriate for good emergency medical services communications EXCEPT:
A. speaking close to the microphone.
B. speaking across or directly into the microphone.
C. talking in a loud voice.
D. speaking without emotion.
E. avoiding the use of slang or profanity.

_____ 130. Repeating an important order to ensure it is understood correctly is:
A. redundancy.
B. multiplexing.
C. the echo procedure.
D. reiteration.
E. either B or D.

_____ 131. The Federal Communications Commission is responsible for all of the following EXCEPT:
A. assigning and licensing radio frequencies.
B. establishing technical standards for radio equipment.
C. monitoring radio frequencies for proper use.
D. formulating acceptable medical information formats.
E. spot-checking radio base stations for proper licensing and records.

Chapter 6: Documentation

_____ 132. The prehospital care report should contain all of the following EXCEPT:
A. a description of your patient's condition when you arrived.
B. a description of your patient's condition after interventions.
C. the medical status of your patient upon arrival at the emergency department.
D. subjective opinions about the patient's dress or actions.
E. all of the above.

_____ 133. Which of the following abbreviations represents patient history?
A. PE
B. HH
C. H
D. Hx
E. A and D

____ 134. Which of the following abbreviations represents alcohol use by the patient?
  A. AOB
  B. ASHD
  C. ETOH
  D. OH+
  E. none of the above

____ 135. Which of the following abbreviations is an indication for administering something as needed?
  A. a.c.
  B. stat
  C. npo
  D. prn
  E. WNL

____ 136. Which of the following is NOT an example of a pertinent negative?
  A. no respiratory distress in an MI patient
  B. nonreactive pupils in a head injury patient
  C. clear breath sounds in a congestive heart failure patient
  D. no history of epilepsy in seizing patient
  E. no pitting edema in a congestive heart failure patient

____ 137. It is better to rephrase a patient's statement regarding history or a symptom, making it more medically correct, than to report it verbatim.
  A. True
  B. False

____ 138. The best time and place to complete the prehospital report form is:
  A. at the scene, if possible.
  B. in the ambulance, en route to the hospital.
  C. at the hospital before you end patient care.
  D. at the hospital after you end patient care.
  E. at the station after the call.

____ 139. The best way to add information to the prehospital care report after it has been submitted to the hospital is to:
  A. search and make changes on all copies.
  B. change only the original report.
  C. create an addendum and add it to all reports.
  D. never add any material to the report once submitted.
  E. make notes only on your personal copy for future reference.

____ 140. The recommended way of making a correction to a prehospital care report is to:
  A. draw a line through the error and initial it.
  B. erase the error completely.
  C. draw up a new form.
  D. blacken the error so it is unreadable.
  E. any of the above.

____ 141. Which of the following is subjective patient information?
  A. mechanism of injury
  B. past medical history
  C. blood pressure
  D. signs of injury
  E. all of the above

____ 142. Which of the following is objective patient information?
  A. chief complaint
  B. past medical history
  C. vital signs
  D. patient description of what happened
  E. all of the above

©2009 Pearson Education, Inc.
Paramedic Care: Principles & Practice, Vol. 2, 3rd. Ed.

_____ 143. The phrase "possible angina" in the assessment management section of a PCR is best described as:
A. the patient's presenting problem.
B. the differential field diagnosis.
C. the field diagnosis.
D. a pertinent negative.
E. both A and C.

_____ 144. Under which element of the SOAP format would you place the patient's chief complaint?
A. subjective
B. objective
C. assessment
D. plan
E. none of the above

_____ 145. Under which element of the SOAP format would you place your field diagnosis?
A. subjective
B. objective
C. assessment
D. plan
E. none of the above

_____ 146. Under which element of the CHART format would you place standing orders?
A. C   D. R
B. H   E. T
C. A

_____ 147. The system of documentation that records information based upon time and sequence of events is the:
A. SOAP format.
B. CHART format.
C. patient management format.
D. call incident approach.
E. either B or D.

_____ 148. When a patient refuses care against your advice, you must be sure to document that:
A. the patient is alert, oriented, and competent to make the decision.
B. you have clearly explained the risks of not receiving care.
C. you have tried to convince the patient to obtain care.
D. you have explained that if the condition worsens the patient should seek immediate care.
E. all of the above.

_____ 149. If you arrive at the scene of a call and are told that your services are not needed, you should:
A. simply return to service, with no need to complete a prehospital care report.
B. simply write "not needed" on the front of the PCR.
C. identify any canceling authority and the time on the PCR.
D. secure the name of the patient as well as any other information, such as the SAMPLE history.
E. all of the above.

_____ 150. Triage tags used for a mass casualty incident usually record:
A. vital patient information.
B. patient priority for care and transport.
C. all minor injuries.
D. hospital destination.
E. both A and B.

SPECIAL PROJECTS

Locating Auscultation Points

On the following illustration, identify where you would locate the stethoscope disk or bell to auscultate breath and heart (pulmonic, aortic, mitral, and tricuspid areas and PMI) sounds.

Fill in the Blanks

Explain the meanings of the following standard medical abbreviations.

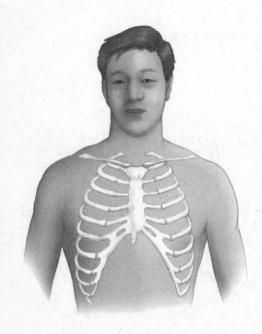

1. CC _____

2. HPI _____

3. SOB _____

4. ASHD _____

5. HBV _____

6. PND _____

7. NTG _____

8. PAL _____

9. CBC _____

10. PMI _____

11. A/O _____

12. p/y _____

13. WNL _____

©2009 Pearson Education, Inc.
Paramedic Care: Principles & Practice, Vol. 2, 3rd. Ed.

14. BVM _____

15. ETT _____

16. NPO _____

17. Rx _____

18. KVO _____

19. SQ _____

20. BBB _____

Crossword Puzzle

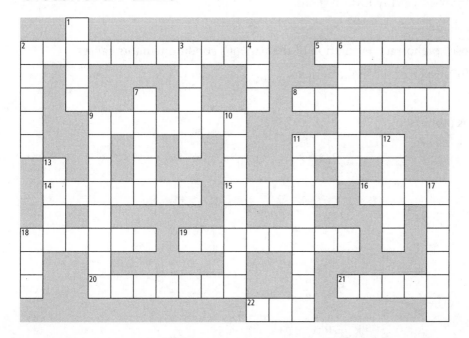

Across

2. Rapid heartbeat

5. Wound

8. High-pitched respiratory sounds

9. Related to the heart

11. _____ complaint: the reason the patient called EMS

14. Fluid build-up in the abdomen

15. Written defamation of another person

16. Type of respirator used when treating a suspected tuberculosis patient

18. Involuntary response to a stimulus

19. Acute alteration in mental function

20. Loud, high-pitched inspiratory wheeze

21. Elements of the head assessment (abbr.)

22. Advanced life support (abbr.)

Down

1. Repeat a verbal order
2. _____ volume: normal respiratory volume
3. Basic EMS communication device
4. Against medical advice (abbr.)
6. Vomitus
7. Sound indicating turbulent blood flow
9. Light, popping, nonmusical inspiratory sounds
10. Type of phone service used by many EMS systems
11. Grating sensation or sound
12. _____ diagnosis; prehospital evaluation of the patient's condition and its causes
13. Questionnaire used for suspected alcoholic patients
17. Severity of an injury or illness
18. Review of the systems (abbr.)

©2009 Pearson Education, Inc.
Paramedic Care: Principles & Practice, Vol. 2, 3rd. Ed.

WORKBOOK ANSWER KEY

Note: Throughout the Answer Key, textbook page references are shown in italics.

Chapter 1: The History

Content Self-Evaluation

MULTIPLE CHOICE

1. D *p. 3*	8. B *p. 5*	15. E *p. 14*
2. A *p. 4*	9. B *p. 8*	16. C *p. 14*
3. A *p. 4*	10. B *p. 9*	17. D *p. 15*
4. C *p. 3*	11. B *p. 11*	18. B *p. 17*
5. A *p. 6*	12. A *p. 11*	19. A *p. 20*
6. C *p. 6*	13. B *p. 12*	20. A *p. 21*
7. C *p. 6*	14. C *p. 14*	

MATCHING

pp. 8–9	*pp. 12–13*	31. O
21. C	26. S	32. R
22. D	27. P	33. T
23. E	28. R	34. Q
24. A	29. Q	35. O
25. B	30. P	

SHORT ANSWER

p. 3

36. The differential field diagnosis is a listing of the primary problems that could cause the chief complaint. The final field diagnosis is the most likely primary problem responsible for the patient's chief complaint, history, and signs and symptoms based upon the patient assessment.

SPECIAL PROJECT: History of the Present Illness

O. (onset of the problem) rapid onset while jogging
P. (provocative/palliative factors) mild pain while deep breathing
Q. (quality of pain) sharp, stabbing
R. (radiation/region of pain) just left of sternum at 3rd intercostal space, with no radiation
S. (severity) 8 on a scale of 1 to 10
T. (time of onset) sudden, with no preceding events
AS. (associated symptoms) none reported
PN. (pertinent negative) denies COPD, asthma, or history of heart problems

Chapter 2: Physical Exam Techniques

Section I

CONTENT SELF-EVALUATION

MULTIPLE CHOICE

1. A *p. 31*	8. A *p. 33*	15. D *p. 44*
2. B *p. 34*	9. C *p. 34*	16. C *p. 45*
3. A *p. 32*	10. B *p. 41*	17. A *p. 45*
4. C *p. 31*	11. C *p. 41*	18. E *p. 45*
5. B *p. 32*	12. A *p. 41*	19. B *p. 45*
6. C *p. 32*	13. E *p. 42*	20. C *p. 45*
7. A *p. 33*	14. A *p. 44*	21. E *p. 46*

22. C *p. 48*	32. B *p. 47*	42. E *p. 61*
23. D *p. 35*	33. E *p. 48*	43. C *p. 62*
24. D *p. 35*	34. D *p. 49*	44. D *p. 63*
25. B *p. 35*	35. B *p. 49*	45. A *p. 69*
26. B *p. 36*	36. D *p. 51*	46. B *p. 69*
27. D *p. 42*	37. E *p. 52*	47. C *p. 73*
28. B *p. 41*	38. A *p. 53*	48. E *p. 73*
29. A *p. 44*	39. B *p. 54*	49. A *p. 77*
30. E *p. 46*	40. D *p. 56*	50. B *p. 83*
31. C *p. 47*	41. E *p. 58*	

SPECIAL PROJECT: Vital Signs

Review pp. 41–48.

Pulse: Evaluate pulse rate, quality (or strength), and rhythm. Pulses should be strong and regular and have a rate of 60 to 100 per minute in adults.

Respirations: Evaluate rate, effort, and quality (depth and pattern). The respiratory rate should be between 12 to 20 times per minute with minimal effort involved in using the diaphragm and intercostal muscles. Breathing should show a regular rhythm and move about 500 mL with each breath.

Blood pressure: Evaluate the diastolic, systolic, and pulse pressures. The normal systolic blood pressure is 100 to 135, the normal diastolic pressure is 60 to 80, and the pulse pressure is between 30 and 40 mmHg. Blood pressures in premenopausal women are slightly lower.

Temperature: Evaluate the core body temperature. The normal core temperature is about 98.6°F, or 37°C.

Section II

MULTIPLE CHOICE

1. B *p. 85*	11. A *p. 93*	21. B *p. 112*
2. D *p. 87*	12. E *p. 94*	22. E *p. 116*
3. B *p. 87*	13. D *p. 94*	23. A *p. 117*
4. E *p. 87*	14. A *p. 95*	24. C *p. 121*
5. B *p. 88*	15. C *p. 98*	25. D *p. 124*
6. A *p. 88*	16. D *p. 101*	26. E *p. 124*
7. C *p. 88*	17. D *p. 103*	27. A *p. 130*
8. C *p. 88*	18. A *p. 104*	28. E *p. 130*
9. B *p. 91*	19. B *p. 111*	29. B *p. 134*
10. D *p. 93*	20. C *p. 111*	30. D *p. 136*

SPECIAL PROJECT: Range of Motion Exercise

Upper Extremity

Joint	Flexion/ Extension	Rotation	Other Motion
Wrist	90/70		(Medial/lateral) 20/45
Elbow	160/0		(Supination/pronation) 90/90
Shoulder	180/50	(Internal/external) 90/90	(Abduction/adduction) 180/75

Lower Extremity

Joint	Flexion/Extension	Rotation	Other Motion
Ankle	Dorsiflex/plantar flex 20/45		(Inversion/eversion) 30/20
Knee	135/90		
Hip	120/0	(External/internal) 40/45	(Abduction) 90

Section III

MULTIPLE CHOICE

1.	C	p. 141	15.	C	p. 154	29.	B	p. 168
2.	A	p. 138	16.	D	p. 154	30.	C	p. 168
3.	D	p. 142	17.	A	p. 157	31.	C	p. 170
4.	E	p. 141	18.	E	p. 156	32.	E	p. 170
5.	E	p. 142	19.	D	p. 157	33.	B	p. 170
6.	E	p. 142	20.	E	p. 157	34.	A	p. 172
7.	A	p. 144	21.	A	p. 157	35.	B	p. 172
8.	E	p. 144	22.	B	p. 160	36.	B	p. 172
9.	B	p. 145	23.	D	p. 161	37.	A	p. 172
10.	C	p. 145	24.	C	p. 159	38.	D	p. 173
11.	D	p. 146	25.	C	p. 164	39.	E	p. 175
12.	D	p. 146	26.	E	p. 167	40.	A	p. 175
13.	B	p. 150	27.	A	p. 168			
14.	A	p. 153	28.	B	p. 168			

MATCHING

See Table 2–11, p. 154.

41.	I, L, M	45.	V, G, X	49.	IX, F, T
42.	II, B, P	46.	VI, D, U	50.	X, I, N
43.	III, H, W	47.	VII, K, Q	51.	XI, E, O
44.	IV, C, S	48.	VIII, A, V	52.	XII, J, R

SPECIAL PROJECT: Auscultation Exercise

CHAPTER 3: Patient Assessment in the Field

Section I

Content Self-Evaluation

MULTIPLE CHOICE

1.	A	p. 186	11.	A	p. 192	21.	A	p. 198
2.	E	p. 186	12.	D	p. 195	22.	E	p. 199
3.	E	p. 187	13.	B	p. 195	23.	C	p. 199
4.	B	p. 188	14.	A	p. 196	24.	A	p. 200
5.	A	p. 188	15.	B	p. 196	25.	C	p. 201
6.	C	p. 189	16.	D	p. 196	26.	A	p. 200
7.	A	p. 189	17.	E	p. 196	27.	B	p. 203
8.	E	p. 190	18.	C	p. 197	28.	D	p. 203
9.	E	p. 190	19.	E	p. 197	29.	A	p. 206
10.	C	p. 191	20.	C	p. 198	30.	C	p. 207

LISTING

p. 186

31. Scene size-up
32. Initial assessment
33. Focused history and physical exam
34. Detailed physical exam
35. Ongoing assessment

SPECIAL PROJECT: Scene Size-Up Exercise

Possible scene hazards include the following:
A. traffic, unstable vehicle, spilled gasoline/fire, stream contamination, unstable/slippery surfaces, hazardous chemicals, broken glass/jagged metal, hot surfaces
B. structural collapse, debris, confined spaces, electrical hazards, explosion, body substances
C. fast water, drowning, hypothermia

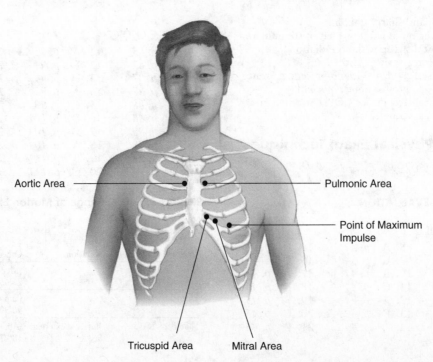

Aortic Area — Pulmonic Area — Point of Maximum Impulse — Tricuspid Area — Mitral Area

MULTIPLE CHOICE

1. C	*p. 211*	11. B	*p. 216*	21. D	*p. 224*
2. D	*p. 211*	12. D	*p. 218*	22. B	*p. 224*
3. B	*p. 212*	13. B	*p. 218*	23. E	*p. 224*
4. A	*p. 213*	14. D	*p. 220*	24. B	*p. 226*
5. E	*p. 214*	15. C	*p. 221*	25. E	*p. 227*
6. A	*p. 214*	16. E	*p. 222*	26. A	*p. 228*
7. D	*p. 214*	17. D	*p. 222*	27. D	*p. 230*
8. A	*p. 214*	18. B	*p. 223*	28. A	*p. 231*
9. B	*p. 215*	19. C	*p. 224*	29. A	*p. 237*
10. C	*p. 216*	20. A	*p. 224*	30. E	*p. 238*

CHAPTER 4: Clinical Decision Making

Content Self-Evaluation

MULTIPLE CHOICE

1. A	*p. 248*	6. C	*p. 250*	11. D	*p. 254*
2. D	*p. 249*	7. A	*p. 250*	12. B	*p. 254*
3. A	*p. 248*	8. B	*p. 250*	13. A	*p. 255*
4. C	*p. 249*	9. B	*p. 250*	14. D	*p. 256*
5. D	*p. 250*	10. A	*p. 250*	15. B	*p. 258*

MATCHING

pp. 256–258

16. B	20. C	23. C
17. D	21. B	24. A
18. A	22. A	25. D
19. A		

CHAPTER 5: Communications

Content Self-Evaluation

MULTIPLE CHOICE

1. E	*p. 264*	10. C	*p. 272*	19. A	*p. 280*
2. B	*p. 266*	11. E	*p. 272*	20. D	*p. 281*
3. C	*p. 266*	12. A	*p. 273*	21. E	*p. 281*
4. E	*p. 268*	13. E	*p. 273*	22. A	*p. 281*
5. D	*p. 269*	14. E	*p. 275*	23. D	*p. 282*
6. B	*p. 269*	15. A	*p. 276*	24. A	*p. 281*
7. A	*p. 270*	16. B	*p. 277*	25. C	*p. 282*
8. D	*p. 271*	17. D	*p. 277*		
9. E	*p. 271*	18. C	*p. 278*		

SPECIAL PROJECT: Documentation: Radio Report/Prehospital Care Report

Your report should include most of the following elements:

Radio message from the scene to medical direction

Unit 89 to Receiving Hospital.

We are at the ball field treating a 13-year-old male who collapsed while playing baseball. He is currently unresponsive to all but painful stimuli, is cool to the touch, and is sweating profusely. Vitals are blood pressure 136/98, pulse 92 and strong, respirations 24 and regular, and pupils equal and slow to react. ECG is showing a normal sinus rhythm. No physical signs of trauma noted, and past medical history is unknown. Oxygen is applied at 12 L via nonrebreather mask. Expected ETA, 20 minutes.

Follow-up radio message to receiving hospital

One IV in left forearm is running TKO with NS. Patient now responding to verbal stimuli. Vitals are blood pressure 134/96, pulse 90 and strong, respirations 24. ECG shows normal sinus rhythm. ETA, 10 minutes.

Ambulance run report form

Please review the accompanying form and check to be sure the form you completed includes the appropriate information. Note that you should include most, if not all, of the information listed on the accompanying sample form. If you have not done this, please review the narrative in the Workbook and determine what is missing from your version. Ensure that no important details are left out of the report.

Review the completed form to ensure that your report includes the appropriate information.

CHAPTER 6: Documentation

Content Self-Evaluation

MULTIPLE CHOICE

1. E	*p. 288*	11. B	*p. 299*	21. E	*p. 303*
2. B	*p. 288*	12. A	*p. 299*	22. D	*p. 304*
3. A	*p. 289*	13. E	*p. 301*	23. E	*p. 304*
4. B	*p. 290*	14. A	*p. 301*	24. A	*p. 305*
5. B	*p. 292*	15. C	*p. 301*	25. E	*p. 303*
6. C	*p. 297*	16. B	*p. 302*	26. B	*p. 305*
7. A	*p. 297*	17. D	*p. 302*	27. A	*p. 306*
8. D	*p. 298*	18. E	*p. 302*	28. D	*p. 307*
9. C	*p. 298*	19. B	*p. 303*	29. E	*p. 308*
10. B	*p. 299*	20. A	*p. 303*	30. C	*p. 309*

MATCHING

pp. 292–296

31. P	40. X	49. F
32. Y	41. M	50. C
33. L	42. J	51. W
34. T	43. Q	52. K
35. A	44. G	53. S
36. E	45. R	54. D
37. B	46. V	55. H
38. O	47. I	
39. U	48. N	

Radio message from the scene to medical direction

Unit 21 to Medical Direction. We are attending a male victim of a one-car crash. He was initially unconscious but is now conscious, alert, and oriented. He has a small contusion on his forehead, the windshield is broken, and there is a small welt on his neck. He was stung by a bee and has had a previous allergic reaction. Vitals are blood pressure 110/76, pulse 90 and strong, respirations 30, and O_2 saturation 94 percent. There are audible wheezes, and he is complaining of "a lump in the throat." He is on 12 L of O_2 via nonrebreather mask and has one IV of LR running TKO. A cervical collar has been applied and spinal immobilization is underway.

Follow-up radio message to community hospital

0.3 mg epinephrine subcutaneously and 50 mg Benadryl IM have been administered. Current vitals are blood pressure 122/78, pulse 68 and strong, respirations 22 and regular, O_2 saturation 98 percent. Breath sounds are now clear. ETA is 10 minutes.

Completed run report for Chapter 5 (page 113).

Ambulance run report form

Please review the accompanying form and check to be sure the form you completed includes the appropriate information. Note that you should include most, if not all, of the information listed on the accompanying sample form. If you have not done this, please review the narrative in the Workbook and determine what is missing from your version. Ensure that no important details are left out of the report.

Review the completed form on the following page to ensure that your report includes the appropriate information.

©2009 Pearson Education, Inc.
Paramedic Care: Principles & Practice, Vol. 2, 3rd. Ed.

Date **Today's Date**	Emergency Medical Services Run Report	Run # **911**

Patient Information

Name: **Thompson, Jim**		
Address: **Unknown**		
City:	St:	Zip:
Age: **13** Birth: / / Sex: [**M**][F]		
Nature of Call: **Unconscious person**		
Chief Complaint: **Unconsciousness—possible heat exhaustion**		

Service Information / Times

Service Information	Times	
Agency: **Unit 89**	Rcvd	**15:15**
Location: **Ball field**	Enrt	**15:16**
Call Origin: **Dispatch**	Scne	**15:22**
Type: Emrg[**X**] Non[ ] Trnsfr[ ]	LvSn	**15:38**
	ArHsp	**15:57**
	InSv	**16:15**

Description of Current Problem:

The patient collapsed while playing baseball on a very hot, sunny

day. Pt. was found to be cool & diaphoretic, unresponsive to

verbal stimuli, and responsive to painful stimuli. Pupils were

normal in size but slow to react. Physical assessment reveals no

apparent signs of trauma or other medical problem.

Medical Problems

Past		Present
[ ]	Cardiac	[ ]
[ ]	Stroke	[ ]
[ ]	Acute Abdomen	[ ]
[ ]	Diabetes	[ ]
[ ]	Psychiatric	[ ]
[ ]	Epilepsy	[ ]
[ ]	Drug/Alcohol	[ ]
[ ]	Poisoning	[ ]
[ ]	Allergy/Asthma	[ ]
[ ]	Syncope	[ ]
[ ]	Obstetrical	[ ]
[ ]	GYN	[ ]

Other: **Unknown**

Trauma Scr: **n/a**   Glasgow: **6**

On-Scene Care: **provided oxygen, removed**

patient from sun and heat. Attempted IV in right

forearm (unsuccessful) started IV in left

forearm w/16 ga NS – TKO

First Aid: **pillow was placed under head**

(removed by EMS)

By Whom? **bystanders**

O$_2$ @ **12** L **15**:27 Via **NRB** | C-Collar **n/a** : | S-Immob. **n/a** | Stretcher **15:37**

Allergies/Meds: **Unknown**

Past Med Hx: **Unknown**

Time	Pulse	Resp.	BP S/D	LOC	ECG
15:27	R: **92** [**X**][i]	R: **24** [s][l]	**136/98**	[a][v][**X**][u]	**Normal Sinus Rhythm**

Care/Comments: **Pt. unresponsive to all but painful stimuli**

15:37	R: **90** [**X**][i]	R: **24** [s][l]	**134/96**	[a][**X**][p][u]	**Normal Sinus Rhythm**

Care/Comments: **Pt. became responsive to verbal stimuli**

15:45	R: **88** [**X**][i]	R: **24** [s][l]	**132/90**	[**X**][v][p][u]	**Normal Sinus Rhythm**

Care/Comments: **Pt. became fully concious, alert, and oriented**

:	R: [r][i]	R: [s][l]	/	[a][v][p][u]	

Care/Comments:

Destination: **Receiving Hospital**	Personnel:	Certification
Reason:[ ]pt [**X**]Closest [ ]M.D. [ ]Other	1. **Your Name**	[**X**][E][O]
Contacted: [**X**]Radio [ ]Tele [ ]Direct	2. **Steve Phillips**	[P][**X**][O]
Ar Status: [**X**]Better [ ]UnC [ ]Worse	3. **n/a**	[P][E][O]

Patient Assessment: Content Review

Content Self-Evaluation

CHAPTER 1: THE HISTORY

1. C	*p. 3*	6. A	*p. 8*	11. E	*p. 15*
2. E	*p. 5*	7. D	*p. 9*	12. C	*p. 16*
3. B	*p. 5*	8. B	*p. 11*	13. B	*p. 18*
4. E	*p. 6*	9. E	*p. 13*	14. D	*p. 21*
5. A	*p. 7*	10. A	*p. 15*	15. B	*p. 24*

CHAPTER 2: PHYSICAL EXAM TECHNIQUES

16. D	*p. 33*	39. B	*p. 63*	62. C	*p. 142*
17. D	*p. 32*	40. D	*p. 70*	63. A	*p. 145*
18. B	*p. 32*	41. E	*p. 77*	64. C	*p. 144*
19. B	*p. 33*	42. A	*p. 85*	65. C	*p. 146*
20. B	*p. 33*	43. D	*p. 87*	66. C	*p. 149*
21. C	*p. 41*	44. D	*p. 88*	67. D	*p. 146*
22. B	*p. 42*	45. A	*p. 88*	68. A	*p. 146*
23. B	*p. 44*	46. D	*p. 90*	69. D	*p. 153*
24. B	*p. 45*	47. D	*p. 94*	70. C	*p. 153*
25. C	*p. 45*	48. D	*p. 95*	71. A	*p. 160*
26. C	*p. 44*	49. E	*p. 98*	72. A	*p. 159*
27. D	*p. 45*	50. A	*p. 101*	73. E	*p. 161*
28. E	*p. 46*	51. E	*p. 109*	74. A	*p. 167*
29. A	*p. 35*	52. E	*p. 112*	75. B	*p. 168*
30. B	*p. 42*	53. B	*p. 112*	76. C	*p. 168*
31. E	*p. 46*	54. A	*p. 117*	77. D	*p. 170*
32. A	*p. 47*	55. B	*p. 122*	78. A	*p. 172*
33. C	*p. 47*	56. E	*p. 130*	79. D	*p. 172*
34. E	*p. 48*	57. D	*p. 130*	80. D	*p. 172*
35. B	*p. 53*	58. A	*p. 134*	81. C	*p. 172*
36. A	*p. 53*	59. D	*p. 141*	82. B	*p. 173*
37. C	*p. 56*	60. C	*p. 138*	83. A	*p. 175*
38. A	*p. 73*	61. E	*p. 142*	84. B	*p. 175*

CHAPTER 3: PATIENT ASSESSMENT IN THE FIELD

85. B	*p. 186*	95. B	*p. 201*	105. A	*p. 220*
86. B	*p. 186*	96. A	*p. 201*	106. B	*p. 222*
87. D	*p. 187*	97. A	*p. 207*	107. E	*p. 222*
88. D	*p. 189*	98. C	*p. 211*	108. C	*p. 223*
89. C	*p. 195*	99. B	*p. 211*	109. D	*p. 224*
90. C	*p. 195*	100. A	*p. 213*	110. C	*p. 224*
91. B	*p. 198*	101. E	*p. 213*	111. C	*p. 228*
92. D	*p. 198*	102. D	*p. 214*	112. C	*p. 230*
93. A	*p. 199*	103. E	*p. 216*	113. B	*p. 231*
94. D	*p. 201*	104. B	*p. 218*		

CHAPTER 4: CLINICAL DECISION MAKING

114. B	*p. 248*	117. E	*p. 251*	120. D	*p. 255*
115. C	*p. 249*	118. A	*p. 253*	121. B	*p. 255*
116. A	*p. 250*	119. C	*p. 254*		

CHAPTER 5: COMMUNICATIONS

122. E	*p. 265*	126. B	*p. 273*	130. C	*p. 282*
123. C	*p. 266*	127. A	*p. 276*	131. D	*p. 282*
124. D	*p. 267*	128. C	*p. 278*		
125. A	*p. 269*	129. C	*p. 281*		

CHAPTER 6: DOCUMENTATION

132. D	*p. 290*	139. C	*p. 301*	146. D	*p. 306*
133. D	*p. 292*	140. A	*p. 301*	147. C	*p. 306*
134. C	*p. 293*	141. B	*p. 302*	148. E	*p. 308*
135. D	*p. 295*	142. C	*p. 303*	149. C	*p. 309*
136. B	*p. 298*	143. E	*p. 304*	150. E	*p. 310*
137. B	*p. 298*	144. A	*p. 305*		
138. D	*p. 301*	145. C	*p. 305*		

©2009 Pearson Education, Inc.
Paramedic Care: Principles & Practice, Vol. 2, 3rd. Ed.

See pp. 89 and 94

Lung sounds: every 5 cm along the midclavicular lines
PMI: 5th intercostal space, left midclavicular line
S1: lower left sternal border
S2: 2nd intercostal space, near sternum

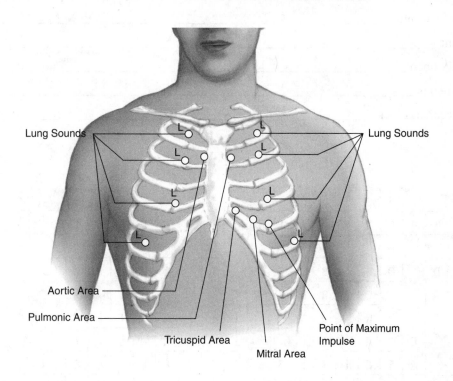

Lung Sounds   Lung Sounds

Aortic Area

Pulmonic Area

Tricuspid Area

Mitral Area

Point of Maximum
Impulse

Fill in the Blanks

See pp. 292–296

1. chief complaint _____

2. history of present illness _____

3. shortness of breath _____

4. atherosclerotic heart disease _____

5. hepatitis B virus _____

6. paroxysmal nocturnal dyspnea _____

7. nitroglycerin _____

8. posterior axillary line _____

9. complete blood count _____

10. point of maximal impulse _____

11. alert and oriented _____

12. pack/years _____

13. within normal limits _____

14. bag-valve mask _____

15. endotracheal tube _____

16. nothing by mouth _____

17. treatment _____

18. keep vein open _____

19. subcutaneous _____

20. bundle branch block _____

```
                 1                                          6
                 E                                  5       L E S I O N
2                           3             4
T A C H Y C A R D I A                     A         L E S I O N
I       H               A           M           M
D       O       7 B     D           A   8 W H E E Z E S
A               9 C A R D I A C   10 C              S
L               R       U       O       E   11 C H I E F   12 F
      13 C      A       I           L       R           S       I
   14 A S C I T E S           15 L I B E L       16 H E P A   17 A
      G         K               U       P           L           C
18 R E F L E X       19 D E L I R I U M       D       U
   O            E                   A       T                   I
   S         20 S T R I D O R       U       21 H E E N T
                         22 A L S                           Y
```